Cystic Fibrosis - Heterogeneity and Personalized Treatment

Edited by Dennis Wat and Dilip Nazareth

Published in London, United Kingdom

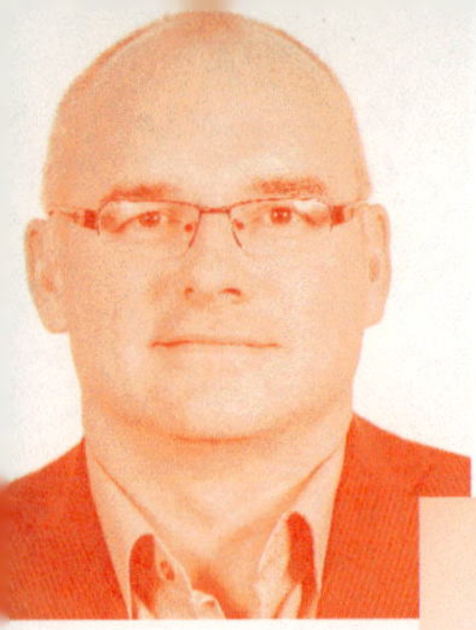
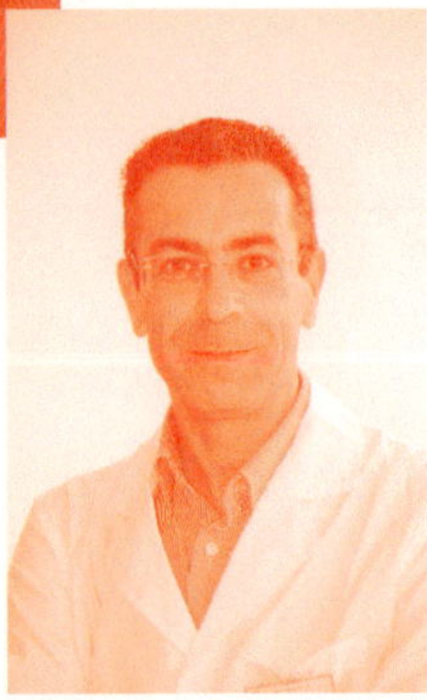
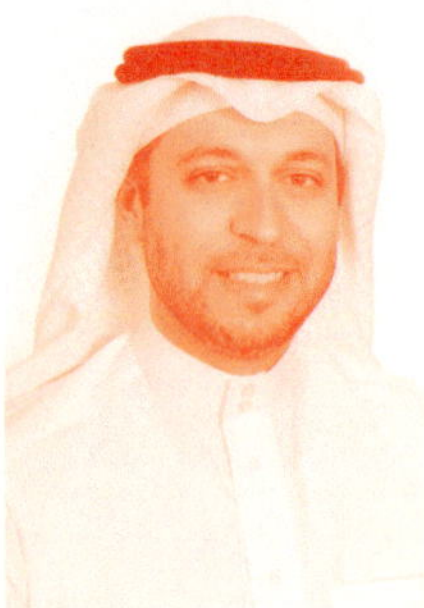
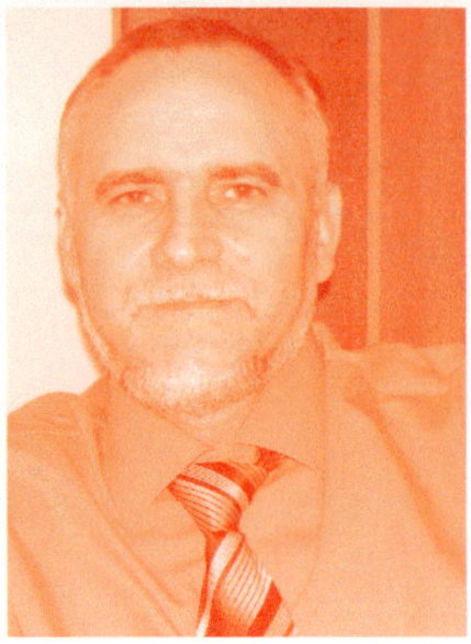
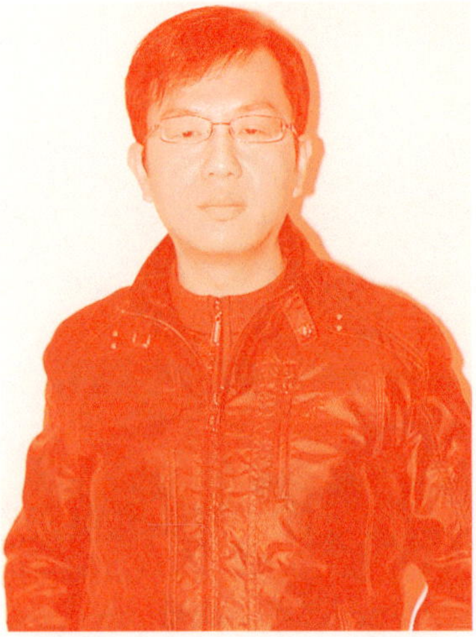
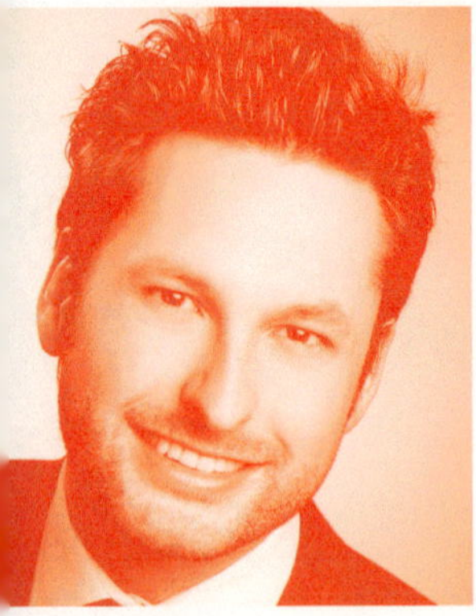
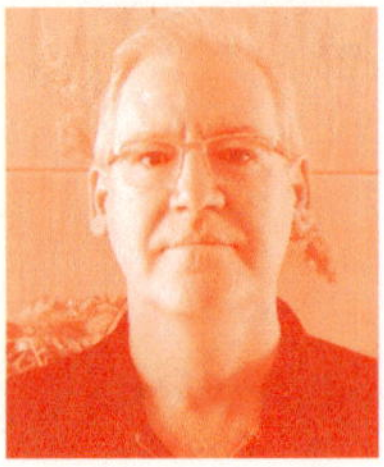

IntechOpen

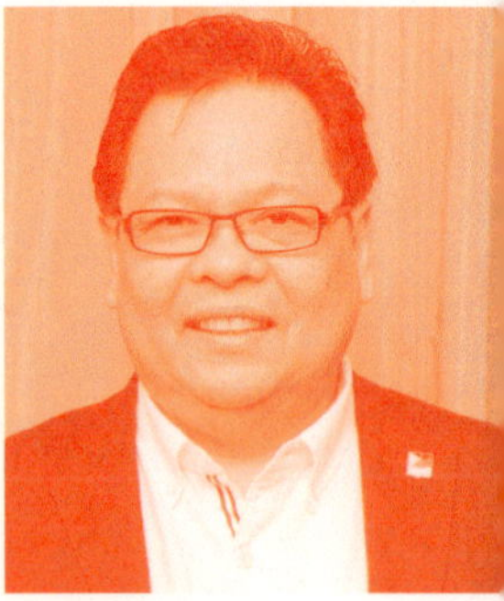
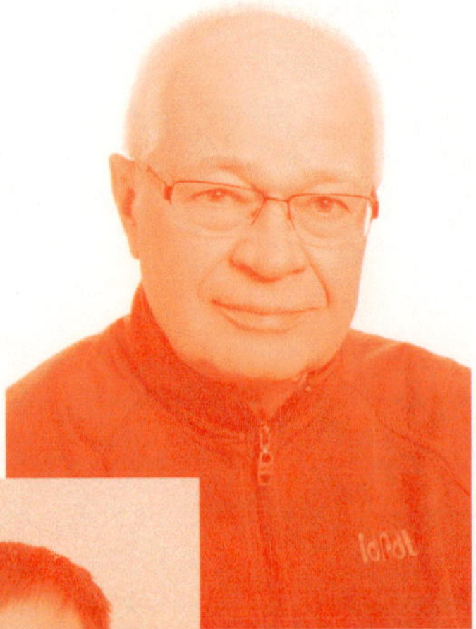
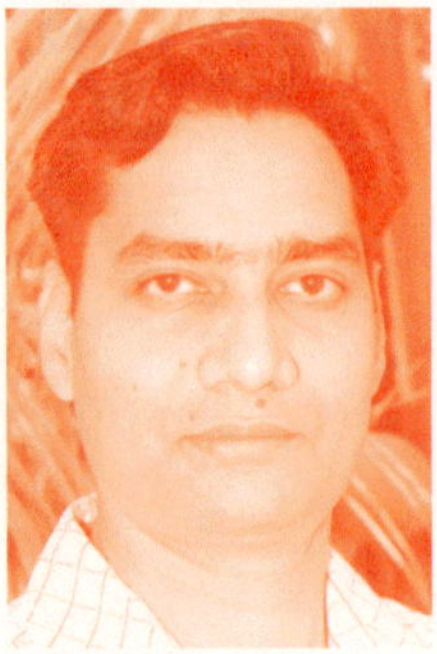
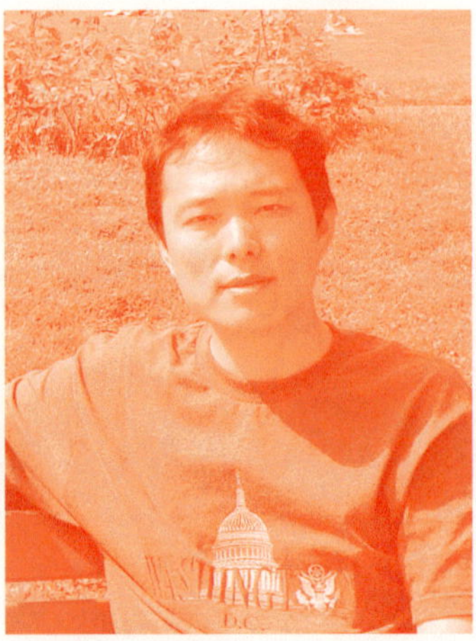
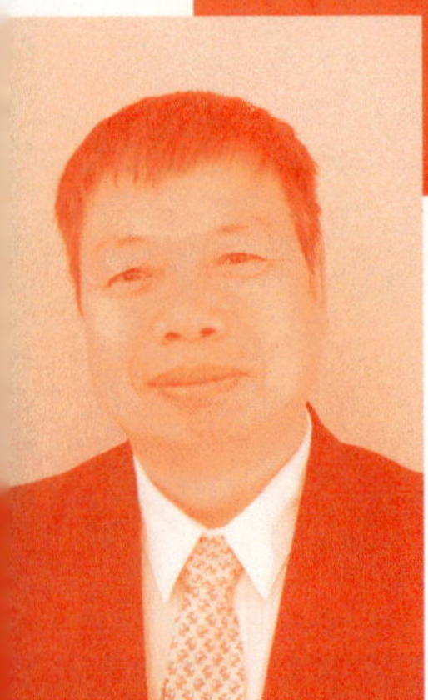
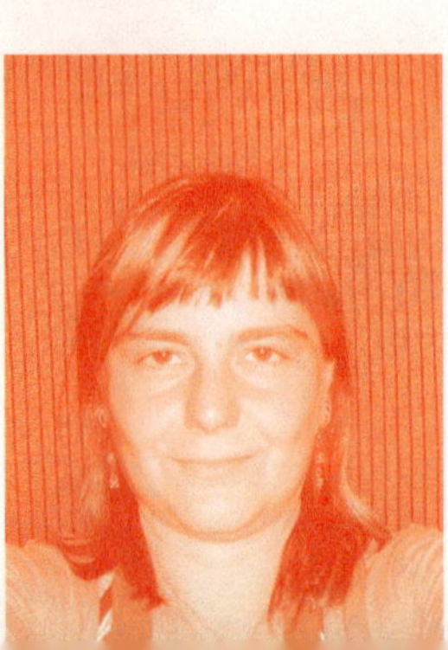

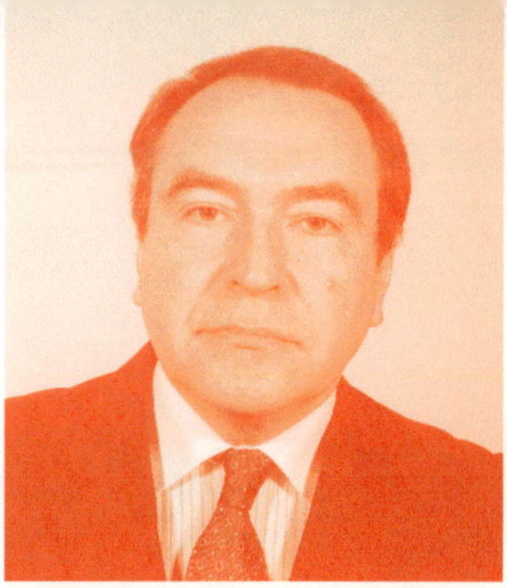
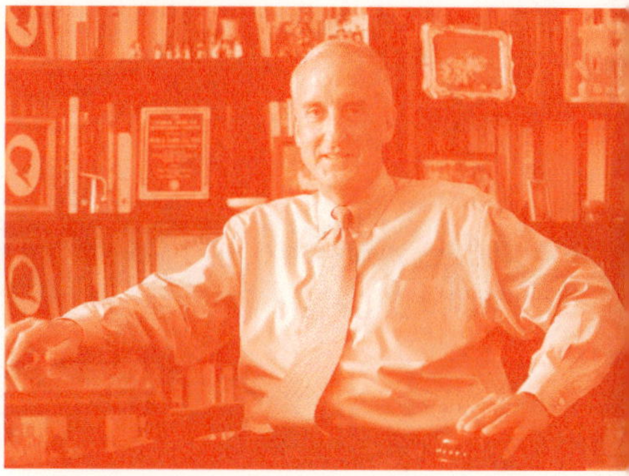
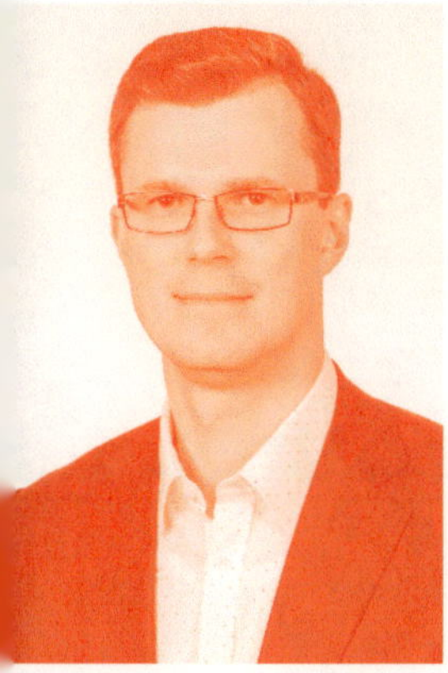
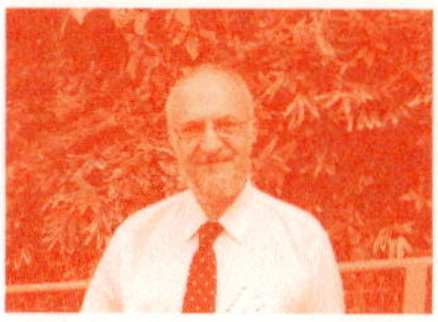
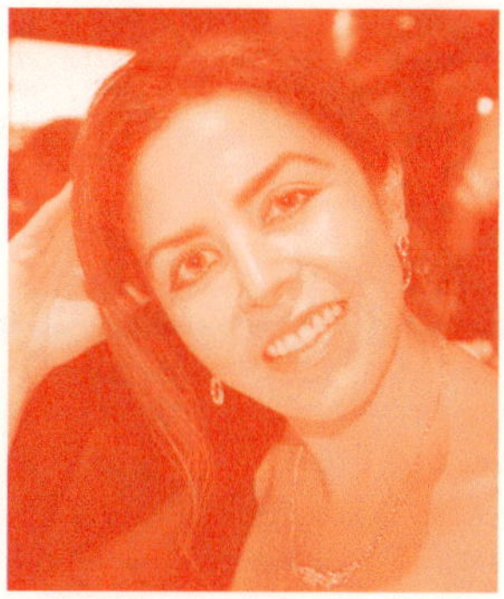

Supporting open minds since 2005

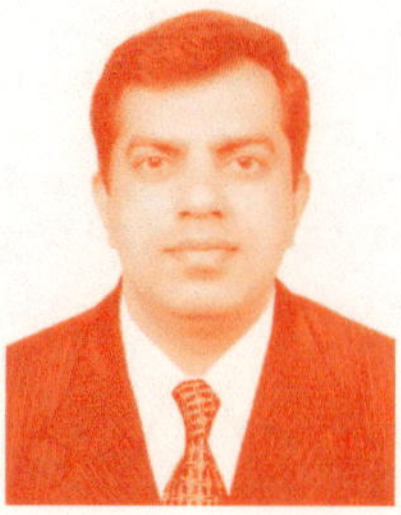
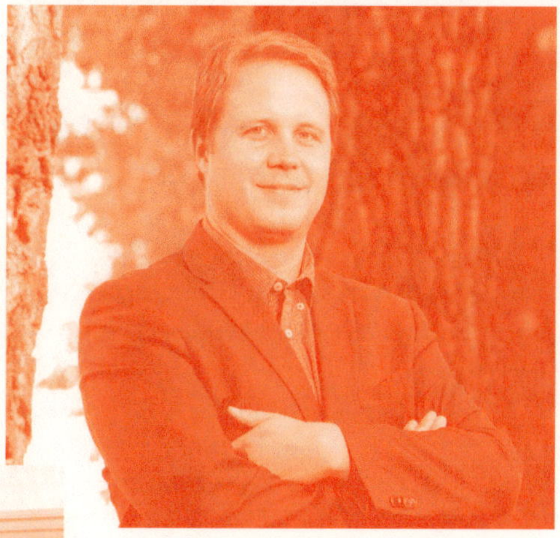
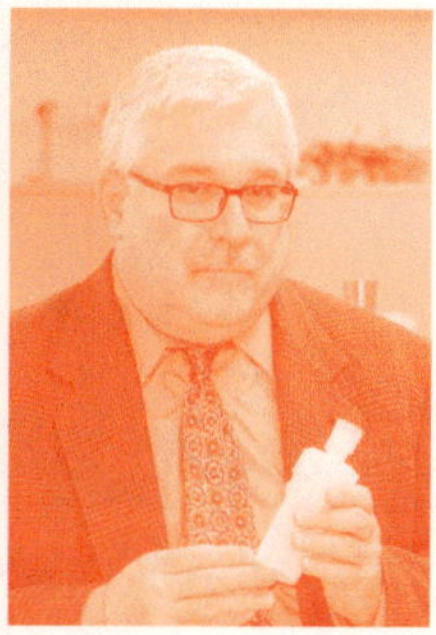
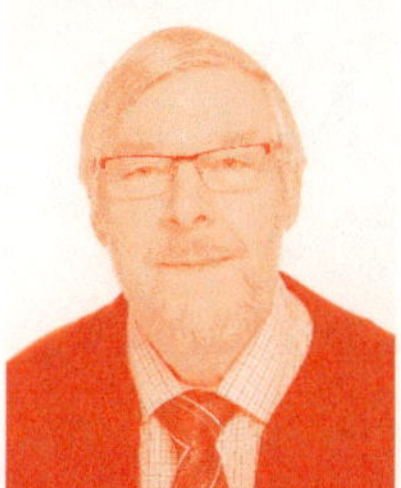
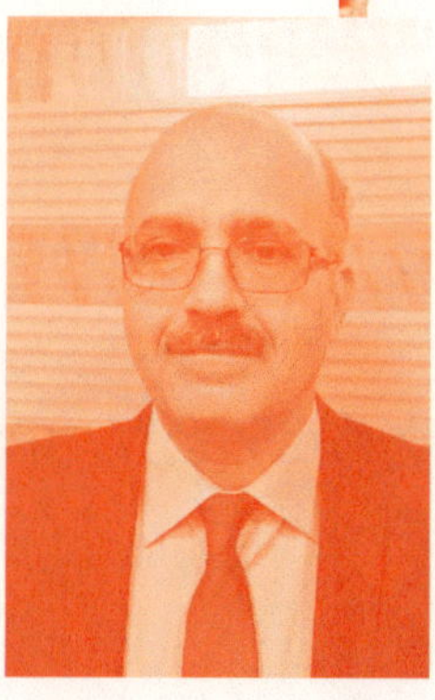
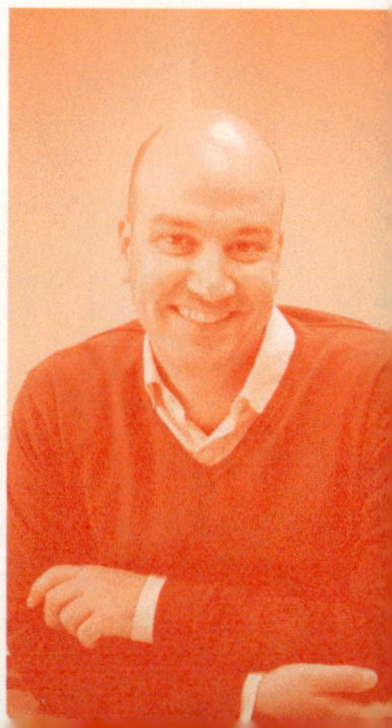
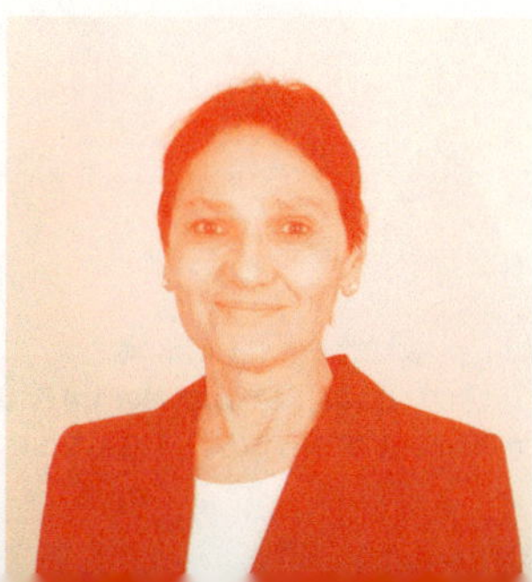

Cystic Fibrosis - Heterogeneity and Personalized Treatment
http://dx.doi.org/10.5772/intechopen.77691
Edited by Dennis Wat and Dilip Nazareth

Contributors
Salah Abdelbary, Rhonda Szczesniak, Bin Huang, Tamara Vagg, Cathy Shortt, Claire Fleming, Mairead McCarthy, Sabin Tabirca, Barry J Plant, Sabina Wiecek, Rita Padoan, Annalisa Fogazzi, Fabianna Timelli, Annalisa Vezzoli, Valentina Tradati, Catherine Rang, John Wilson, Tom Kotsimbos, Dennis Wat, Freddy J Frost, Dilip Nazareth

First published in London, United Kingdom, 2020 by IntechOpen
IntechOpen is the global imprint of INTECHOPEN LIMITED, registered in England and Wales, registration number: 11086078, 7th floor, 10 Lower Thames Street, London, EC3R 6AF, United Kingdom
Printed in Croatia

British Library Cataloguing-in-Publication Data
A catalogue record for this book is available from the British Library

Additional hard and PDF copies can be obtained from orders@intechopen.com

Cystic Fibrosis - Heterogeneity and Personalized Treatment
Edited by Dennis Wat and Dilip Nazareth
p. cm.
Print ISBN 978-1-78984-145-9
Online ISBN 978-1-78984-146-6
eBook (PDF) ISBN 978-1-83880-968-3

For EU product safety concerns:
IN TECH d.o.o., Prolaz Marije Krucifikse Kozulić 3, 51000 Rijeka, Croatia, info@intechopen.com or visit our website at intechopen.com.

Meet the editors

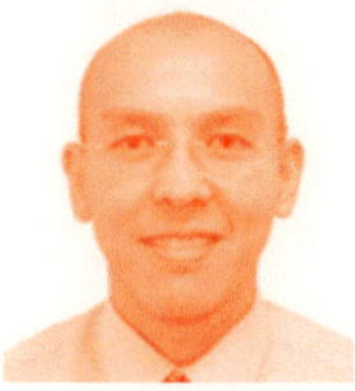

Dennis Wat, MD, obtained his undergraduate degree (MB BCh) in 1998 in Cardiff, UK. In 2007, he was awarded an MD from the University of Cardiff where he researched the impact of respiratory viruses in cystic fibrosis (CF). In 2009, he was appointed as Respiratory Consultant in the Adult CF Unit at Papworth Hospital, Cambridge, UK. In 2012, he moved to Liverpool, UK to join the respiratory community and Liverpool Adult CF services. Apart from CF, Dr. Wat has vast experience in the management of COPD, bronchiectasis, asthma and oxygen therapy in the management of chronic lung diseases. He has published widely in pulmonary medicine, including papers in peer-reviewed journals and book chapters. He is a principal investigator in a number of clinical trials.

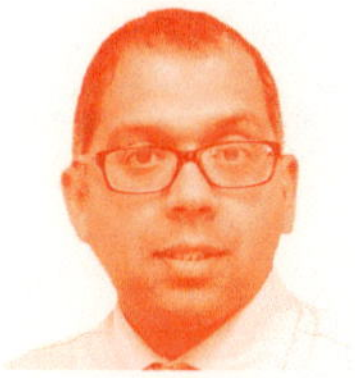

Dr Dilip Nazareth became interested in a career in cystic fibrosis after training as a Junior Doctor at the Royal Brompton Hospital in London. He subsequently undertook his higher training posts in respiratory and general medicine in Merseyside. He spent a further 2 years as a Clinical and Research Fellow at the prestigious Adult Cystic Fibrosis (CF) Unit at Liverpool Heart and Chest Hospital, which is among the largest CF units in the country. During this time, he carried out research on Cystic Fibrosis Related Diabetes (CFRD), and completed his (Doctoral) MD thesis through the University of Liverpool. Following completion of his training, he worked as a consultant in CF, respiratory and general medicine at University Hospitals Bristol NHS Trust, prior to relocating back to Merseyside. His research interests are in CFRD, CF renal disease, CF microbiology and CF antibiotics. He has published several scientific articles in respiratory medicine and CF and continues to undertake research. He previously was a Research Affiliate at the National Institute for Health - Research Biomedical Research (University of Bristol) and a member of the British Thoracic Society CF Specialist Advisory Group. He is also an International Examiner and Examination Chair for the postgraduate medical examinations of the Royal College of Physicians, London.

Contents

Preface

Cystic fibrosis (CF) is one of the most common fatal inherited diseases. The discovery of the cystic fibrosis transmembrane conductance regulator (CFTR) gene 30 years ago set the cornerstone for unravelling the pathogenesis of CF lung disease, continuous development of disease-modifying agents, and the inception of mutation-specific therapies, which are now becoming available for a subgroup of patients.

This book provides an update on aspects of CF lung disease. Frost et al. describe the use of novel culture-independent techniques such as next-generation sequencing to analyse the lung microbiome, allowing us to further understand the diversity, complexity, and effects of acute exacerbations, and the use of antibiotics on bacterial communities. The understanding of the CF microbiome presents new opportunities for disease management in CF and has the potential to explore the impact of CFTR modulators. Abdelbary also provides an overview of the microbiology in CF including the impact of bacterial colonisation, fungi and respiratory viruses.

The overview of CFTR modulators and gene therapy provides understanding of personalized therapeutic options with a focus on an individual's specific mutations. Rang et al. provide a succinct summary of these exciting treatment modalities in CF and how these treatment modalities for forever alter the care of these patients.

Szczesniak et al. discuss the use of CF registries that have the potential to improve on CF clinical management effectiveness and the development of treatment policies, although missing and confounding data can be huge challenges in the evolution of these policies.

Around 40 percent of patients with CF have some form of liver abnormalities. In recent years, an increase in CF-related liver disease (CFLD) has been noted. This is most likely related to patients with CF who are being screened more stringently for liver disease starting from a young age. Wiecek et al. provide an overview of the risk factors, clinical symptoms, diagnostic methods and treatment of liver changes in the course of CF.

In light of COVID-19, many health-governing bodies are turning to remote consultations in order to minimise the risk of infection for staff and patients. Fogazzi et al. describe the use of video education to improve the adherence of airway clearance and inhaled therapies. This is an important stress test depicting the usefulness of technology in this specific patient cohort.

Finally, Vagg et al. describe the design and development of a patient passport mHealth application for adults with CF. This application allows patients access to their own data. It will be of benefit when travelling abroad and between CF centres. This technology also has the potential to improve the quality and safety of care.

This book is invaluable for clinicians, scientists and researchers involved in the care of patients with CF.

Dennis Wat
Consultant Chest Physician,
Adult Cystic Fibrosis Unit,
Liverpool Heart and Chest Hospital,
Liverpool, UK

Honorary Senior Clinical Lecturer,
University of Liverpool,
UK

Dilip Nazareth
Consultant Chest Physician,
Adult Cystic Fibrosis Unit,
Liverpool Heart and Chest Hospital,
Liverpool, UK

Honorary Senior Lecturer,
Institute of Infection and Global Health,
University of Liverpool,
UK

Chapter 1

The Pulmonary Microbiome in Cystic Fibrosis

Freddy J. Frost, Dilip Nazareth and Dennis Wat

Abstract

The chronic colonisation of the lower airways by bacterial pathogens is the leading cause of morbidity and mortality in patients with cystic fibrosis (CF). The use of novel culture-independent techniques such as next-generation sequencing (NGS) to analyse the lungs has allowed us to further understand the diversity, the complexity, the effects of acute exacerbations and the use of antibiotics on the bacterial communities. The understanding of the CF microbiome to airway disease remains a fascinating area of research; it presents new opportunities for disease management in CF and has the potential to explore the effects of cystic fibrosis transmembrane conductance regulator (CFTR) modulators. It also allows further appreciation regarding the roles played by anaerobic organisms within the CF airways. It is also of interest that a number of studies have demonstrated that the fluctuations of microbiome are not necessarily associated with the patient's clinical status. Despite the available evidence, there remain many challenges that must be overcome if microbiome profiling is going to influence future clinical practice. The effects of fungus and the emergence of nontuberculous mycobacteria in CF are also briefly discussed in this chapter.

Keywords: cystic fibrosis, microbiome, CFTR modulators, nontuberculous mycobacteria, *Aspergillus*

1. Introduction

Traditional culture techniques rely on growing bacteria on media in laboratory conditions often optimised for growth of specific organisms so that they can then subsequently be identified. In the last 20 years, novel techniques utilising next-generation sequencing (NGS) to identify bacteria have become available, enabling detection and description of bacterial communities without the need for conventional culture. These technologies have allowed a greater understanding of bacterial communities throughout the human body and have revealed functional roles in both health and disease.

A healthy human gut, for example, is home to a highly diverse community of bacteria, termed as microbiome, which has symbiotic functions including metabolism of otherwise indigestible compounds and defence against opportunistic pathogens [1, 2]. Furthermore, bacteria in the gut influence the stimulation and development of the innate mucosal immune system [3]. In addition to the roles in health, there has been significant interest in the relationship between microbiomes and diseases such as obesity, inflammatory bowel disease and diabetes mellitus [4–6].

Studies utilising culture-independent techniques to analyse the lungs have identified the presence of bacterial communities that are much more complex than the previously appreciated. The lungs were long considered to be an inherently sterile environment, in part due to the fact that conventional culture techniques often yielded negative results during health and it was only during disease that pathogens were detected. However, the advent of culture-independent techniques has demonstrated that multiple organisms comprise a community, termed the 'microbiome', in the lungs of patients, both healthy and diseased [7–9]. In this chapter, we discuss the techniques employed in 16S rRNA sequencing and the evidence these techniques have generated so far in relation to cystic fibrosis.

2. 16S rRNA gene sequencing

The 16S rRNA gene codes for a ribosomal subunit present in nearly all bacteria. The gene itself is approximately 1.5 kb long and consists of conserved regions, similar in nearly all microorganisms, and nine variable regions labelled, V1–V9, which are practically specific to each microorganism [10]. The identification of a specific DNA sequence that corresponds to the known variable region of 16S rRNA gene can allow discrimination of the presence and relative abundance of different microorganisms (**Figure 1**).

Once the samples have been processed, DNA is extracted, and the 16S rRNA gene is amplified using polymerase chain reaction (PCR). Next-generation sequencing allows elucidation of the precise gene sequences, and online reference databases can then be used to match each sequence to an organism and quantify its relative proportion within a multispecies population. However, it is important to note that sequencing of the 16S rRNA gene has limited resolution and often cannot distinguish species with similar gene sequences apart. Therefore, instead of distinct species, sequences are referenced against and assigned into operational taxonomic units (OTU) (see **Table 1**).

Given the large number of species identified even in healthy lungs, ecological theory and analyses are often employed to understand community dynamics [9]. According to ecological principles, the composition of the lung microbiome is determined by three factors:

1. Immigration of organisms into the lung

2. Elimination of microbes from the airways

3. Regional growth factors [11]

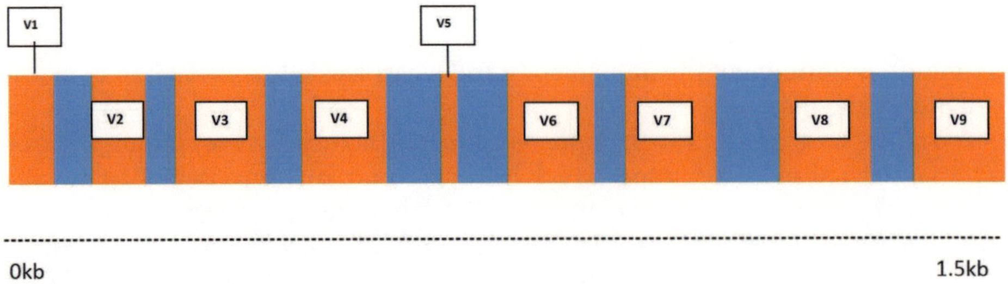

Figure 1.
Schematic illustration of structure of the 16S rRNA gene. Orange regions—variable regions; blue region—conserved region.

Term	Definition
Microbiome	The microorganisms in a particular environment
16S rRNA gene	A gene which codes for a ribosomal subunit. Present in all prokaryotes and has variable regions, which differ slightly between bacterial species
Richness	A measure of the number of species in a community
Evenness	A measure of similarity of the relative abundance for each species in a community That is, does one species dominate, or do all species have similar relative abundance?
Diversity	A measure of variety in a community. Combination of richness and evenness
Alpha diversity	Within-sample diversity
Beta diversity	Between-sample diversity
Operational taxonomic unit (OTU)	Group of strains/species with similar 16S rRNA gene sequences

Table 1.
Glossary of terms and definitions.

The lung microbiome in healthy individuals is dictated largely by immigration and elimination and hence generally consists predominantly of those Gram-negative anaerobes also resident in the oral flora such as *Prevotella* and *Veillonella* spp. [11]. However, in disease the regional growth conditions are altered, and niches for other species to thrive are created. In CF, for example, viscous secretions, altered pH, nutrient availability and architectural disturbance may all help select for a community of altered composition to that of healthy individuals. How this community changes over time, in response to the intensive antibiotic treatment that people with CF are exposed to, has been the subject of much interest in the last decade.

3. CF respiratory microbiota in early life

Understanding the development of the CF respiratory microbiota in early life has attracted interest in order to appreciate the driving factors behind the distinct microbiota seen later in life and also to identify potential opportunities for intervention. Neonates and infants cannot expectorate sputum independently, and bronchoalveolar lavage (BAL) is only used sparingly; hence, upper respiratory tract samples are often used as surrogates. The imperfection of this approach was recently highlighted where large differences in concordance between BAL samples and upper respiratory tract (URT) samples were observed in some taxa [12]. Nevertheless, concordance was high for some important taxa such as *Moraxella* and *Staphylococcus,* and in the absence of less invasive techniques, URT sampling enables early estimation of the neonatal lower respiratory tract.

The composition of CF nasopharyngeal microbiota diverges from that of non-CF infants as early as the first few months of life [13, 14]. Newborn healthy infants appear to have nasopharyngeal microbiota dominated by *Moraxella* spp., *Corynebacterium spp.* and *Haemophilus* spp., a community structure that persists for at least the first 6 months of life. Conversely the CF nasopharynx microbiome is initially dominated by *Staphylococcus aureus* before a gradual increase in *Streptococcus* spp. and *Moraxellaceae* at 3 months of age [13]. Despite the increased *S. aureus* seen in CF, there were no decreases in measures of richness or diversity indicating that changes are due to differing microenvironment rather than interspecies competition [15].

The divergence observed in the first few months of life usually precedes antibiotic administration and demonstrates that CF itself is associated with compositional changes in the microbiota, but as CF infants grow older, exposure to antibiotics, either via acute treatment for respiratory illnesses or prophylaxis against classic CF pathogens, becomes inevitable. Mika et al. investigated the relationship between antibiotics and the nasal microbiota by prospectively following 30 newborn infants with CF with fortnightly sampling for the first 12 months of life [14]. Antibiotic administration was associated with an increase in the Shannon diversity measure (a measure of the richness and evenness of a community), but this was judged to be most likely secondary to an increase in transient colonisers. Interestingly, antibiotic therapy was staphylococcal directed, but decreases in *Staphylococcus* OTUs were not seen. Instead significant reductions in *Moraxellaceae* were observed, and when oligotyping was used to observe changes in *Staphylococcus* at the species level, mild reductions in *S. aureus* were offset by increases in *S. epidermidis*, leading the authors to suggest that *S. epidermidis* may act as a reservoir of resistance. These findings were supported by Prevaes et al. who conducted a similar study in a slightly older population (mean age 2 years old) [13]. Antibiotic treatment was observed to be associated with reductions in *Moraxellaceae* and *S. aureus* OTUs, with increases in other staphylococcal OTUs, although more specific oligotyping was not performed.

As babies grow older, sampling from the lower airways becomes more common, and comparisons between the lower and upper airways become feasible. Given the close proximity and interrelated spaces of the nose, throat and lungs, it could be expected that they all may share similar community structures; however, the reality is that the nasal community appears different from that of the throat and lung, which are much more closely aligned. Boutin et al. found differences in the community structure of the nasal cavity compared to throat and sputum samples; in that diversity, richness and evenness were significantly higher in nasal samples, and up to 21 of the 76 most abundant nasal OTUs were not present in the throat or sputum samples [16]. Interestingly, the authors also found that subjects could be broadly defined into one of two ecotypes based on the presence or absence of *Pseudomonas*, and the similarities between throat and sputum samples began to diminish once *Pseudomonas* was present. Muhlebach et al. supported these findings in a recently published study, which for the first time included routine sequential BAL sampling in young children as part of the large AREST-CF cohort in Australia and the USA. They showed that lower airway cultures mirrored that of the oral cavity until approximately age 2, when increasing predominance of known CF pathogens was observed and communities diverged [17]. This has a number of clinical implications in that, firstly, throat swabs can provide adequate representation of the lower airways in very young children and, secondly, prevention or delay of this transition point by manipulation of the microbiota could theoretically be a strategy to improve outcomes later in life.

4. Progressive loss of diversity

Once the lungs are colonised with CF pathogens, a pattern of progressively uneven community structures ensues. Cox et al. examined biobanked sputum samples from a cohort of 63 clinically stable people with CF of ages ranging from 9 months to 72 years [7]. This cross-sectional approach identified the loss of community richness, evenness and diversity as age increased. *Pseudomonas* and *Burkholderia* OTUs began to progressively dominate in older subjects, and the changes in community structure were inversely associated with pulmonary function. In a similar study design with 269 patients, Coburn et al. also found sample diversity inversely correlated with age and disease stage. Progressive loss of diversity was particularly correlated with *Pseudomonas* and *Burkholderia* abundance, which notably increased after the age of 25 [18].

Zhao et al. were the first to confirm these findings longitudinally when they followed up six patients over a 9-year period with serial sputum collections. It was observed that the three patients with what they termed as more 'progressive' disease had significant decreases in community diversity over the course of several years. Decreasing lung function and increasing age were also associated with decreasing community diversity [19]. This study was soon followed by Fodor et al. who focussed more on changes in the microbiota associated with acute changes in clinical status but did observe a strong correlation between low species richness and poor lung function [20]. Stokell et al. followed up a single patient up to over 3 years and observed increasing total bacterial load as well as diminishing community richness and diversity [21].

Contrastingly, Whelan et al. recently published a study of six patients who submitted thrice-weekly sputum samples for a year [22]. No overall changes in community structure were observed over the course of the year, and the authors concluded that the respiratory microbiome is unique to each patient and the previously reported associations between community structure and clinical parameters may be true on a cohort/population level but not at an individual level. There is some merit in this argument, but it is also worth noting that the six patients in the study appeared relatively stable with a median of only one exacerbation in the 12-month study period. It is also therefore a possibility that the follow-up period was not long enough to capture the more indolent changes likely to be present in those patients [23]. A much longer study period was adopted by Acosta et al. [24] who analysed samples from matched patients with biobanked sputum samples in three historic cohorts spanning nearly 20 years at a single centre. Across all the three cohorts, the core microbiome constituents were preserved, but the proportion of *Pseudomonas*-dominated communities was reduced, and overall diversity increased in the more recent cohorts. Community structure improved gradually from the most historic cohort to the most recent, and these changes appeared to correlate with the generally improving clinical status of people with CF, confirming the previously described observed association between community structure and clinical outcomes [24].

The association reported in most studies between community structure and clinical outcomes has inevitably led to the question of whether a less diverse or even rich microbiome is simply a marker of increased pulmonary disease or is itself a driver in disease pathogenesis [25]. If the latter were true, efforts to promote a more diverse community could have the potential to slow pulmonary disease progression. An Italian group has led efforts to find patterns or signatures in the microbiome that may predispose patients to accelerated lung function decline; however, no causal association has been elucidated [26–28]. Instead, Zhao et al. found that the relationship between age, lung function and community diversity disappeared once controlled for antibiotic use, thus suggesting antibiotic therapy is the predominant driver of reducing community diversity [19]. The same group later developed a statistical approach to more precisely correct the antibiotic exposure when examining relationships between microbiota and clinical outcomes. The approach was applied to 478 sputum samples and confirmed that antibiotic use was an independent predictor for decreased diversity [29].

Accurately recording antibiotic use is troublesome in longitudinal studies due to the frequent episodic use of antibiotics in CF which is often self-directed by patients themselves, due to the widespread use of long-term antibiotics for which compliance may be heterogeneous and also due to the retrospective nature of a number of CF microbiome studies [30]. However, Pittman et al. were able to prospectively perform bronchoscopy and record antibiotic exposure of 32 subjects as part of the AREST-CF study. In that study, community diversity was much lower in the BAL of those patients receiving antibiotics [31].

Thus it appears likely that the strong association between community structure and degree of lung disease is related to the inevitable prolonged and aggressive use of antibiotics in CF rather than direct pathogenesis from a less diverse microbiome.

5. Community changes with acute pulmonary exacerbations

Despite the importance of exacerbations on long-term outcomes of people with CF, the pathophysiology of these events remains undefined [32, 33]. Clinically, exacerbations are frequent and are characterised by rapid changes in symptoms such as an increase in sputum volume or purulence, shortness of breath and fatigue. The precise mechanisms underlying these important events remain elusive, and studies looking for answers using culture-independent techniques have not found consistent answers. For example, one may expect to find evidence of increases in known pathogens at the time of exacerbations, yet there is no consistent evidence of this [23]. In fact, a number of studies have found the CF microbiota to be extremely stable over time and resilient to change at exacerbation and following subsequent treatment [19, 20, 34, 35].

However, when the community structure as a whole is considered, a number of larger studies have found reduced diversity or richness at the times of exacerbation compared to clinical stability. Coburn et al. found small decreases in Shannon diversity in exacerbation samples compared to their baseline study of 269 people with CF [18]. Similarly, Filkins et al. found that samples taken during exacerbations had significantly lower diversity than samples taken when patients were stable [36]. Perhaps most convincingly, Li et al. collated data from 18 previous studies to analyse over 700 sputum samples and found that there were significant reductions in community richness at exacerbation [37].

Whilst increases in *P. aeruginosa* at the time of exacerbation have not been seen consistently, they have been observed in some cases. Carmody et al. followed up four patients for 3 months with daily sputum sampling and observed daily stability between exacerbations but increased *P. aeruginosa* abundance at the time of exacerbation in some patients and increases in *Prevotella* in others [38]. These findings help introduce two new concepts: firstly, the potential for exacerbations to appear similar phenotypically but have different underlying aetiology with only some being due to changes that can be observed in the microbiota and, secondly, that previously overlooked anaerobes may play a pathogenic role.

The first concept is supported by Whelan et al. who found in longitudinal sampling of six patients that some but not all exacerbations were associated with changes in the microbiota [22]. Attempts to identify different types of exacerbations in COPD have identified four distinct aetiological clusters, bacterial, viral, eosinophilic predominant and 'paucinflammatory', and even though these clusters may not be mirrored in CF, it is plausible that not all exacerbation clusters would be associated with changes apparent in either individual taxa or overall bacterial community structure [39].

Changes in the metabolic activity of specific taxa or the community as a whole triggering an exacerbation could be another explanation for an apparent lack of change in the community structure seen in some studies. The metabolites lactate and putrescine were found by Twomey et al. to increase during exacerbation in the absence of clear changes in the community structure [40]. Quinn et al. used the ecological functional networking to identify the non-mevalonate pathway of isoprenoid synthesis as a 'keystone' pathway in CF infections. Intriguingly fosmidomycin, an antimalarial agent, is known to be effective at targeting this pathway [41].

The second concept to emerge from the study of Carmody et al. relates to the changes in *Prevotella* abundance at the time of exacerbation and raises the prospect that species not considered conventional CF pathogens may play a role in exacerbations [42]. Anaerobic species are easily overlooked in conventional selective culturing due to the requirement for anoxic culture yet are identified frequently in culture-independent analyses of the CF lower airways. In addition to *Gemella*, both *Prevotella* and *Streptococcus anginosus (milleri)* have been found to have associations with clinical stability [36, 38, 42]. Anaerobes have been shown to have the potential to modulate *P. aeruginosa* gene expression in the polymicrobial setting; hence, even if they are not directly pathogenic, they may still play a contributory role to the pathogenesis of some exacerbations [43, 44].

To summarise, the aetiologies underpinning the transition from a stable state to an acute exacerbation are not well understood. It is likely that there multiple aetiological clusters but only some of which may be associated with changes in community structure.

6. Community changes associated with treatment for acute pulmonary exacerbations

Traditional dogma would dictate that intensive, targeted antimicrobial therapy with dual anti-pseudomonal agents will result in significant reductions in abundance of *P. aeruginosa*; however, in a similar vein to the findings from studies of the onset of exacerbations, microbiota responses to treatment for acute pulmonary exacerbations in CF have not aligned with this conventional understanding of infections.

One of the predominant themes that has emerged from studies of the respiratory microbiota response to acute antibiotics is that *P. aeruginosa* is not impacted to the same degree as other members of the community. For example, Daniels et al. studied 12 adult CF subjects across the cycle of an exacerbation and treatment and found that following initiation of anti-pseudomonal antimicrobials, the relative abundance of *P. aeruginosa* actually increased, alongside a reduction in the total number of species detected [45]. Cuthbertson et al. also found no evidence of reduced *P. aeruginosa* abundance in a study of 12 CF patients receiving treatment for pulmonary exacerbations [45]. Instead, reductions in *Streptococcus sanguinis*, *Prevotella* and *Porphyromonas* OTUs were observed [35]. Similarly, Li et al., in their analysis of over 700 sputum samples, found that antibiotic treatment had no effect on *Pseudomonas* abundance but did have significant effects on *Gemella*, *Staphylococcus*, *Actinomyces, Moraxellaceae* and *Fusobacterium* [37]. Further, Fodor et al. again found that dominant taxa such as *Pseudomonas* and *Burkholderia* were unchanged when compared at the beginning and end of an exacerbation but the relative abundances of *Gemella, Streptococcus* and a small number of other less abundant OTUs were all reduced [20].

In contrast, two studies have found reductions in *P. aeruginosa* following treatment. Firstly, Zemanick et al. investigated the association between inflammation and changes to the airway microbiota during treatment for exacerbations and found that although bacterial load did not change, the relative abundance of *P. aeruginosa* was observed to decrease and that these changes correlated with improved lung function [46]. A reduction in *P. aeruginosa* abundance following treatment was also reported by Smith et al., who noted rapid decreases in *P. aeruginosa* abundance and an associated increase in diversity following the initiation of intravenous antibiotic treatment for pulmonary exacerbations in CF, although these changes were transient and returned to baseline following the completion of treatment [47].

There are a number of factors that may explain the differences between the studies mentioned in this section, and many of them apply to studies of the CF microbiome in general. The most obvious is the heterogeneous study designs, which are mostly retrospective and observational in nature and include a wide range of antibiotic regimens. For example, some authors such as Cuthbertson and Daniels included exacerbations treated with oral antibiotics as well as those requiring intravenous therapy [35, 45]. Milder exacerbations are often treated with oral antibiotics, and hence associated changes in the microbiota may also be expected to be more subtle. Even in those studies where only intravenous regimens were used, the antibiotic regimens or doses given are often not listed. The lack of a control or comparator group further makes interpreting results difficult [35, 45].

A further consideration is the sampling timeframes in each study, where again there exists a considerable variation that may have implications for interpreting results, particularly given that Smith et al. reported significant but transient reductions in *P. aeruginosa* abundance in the first few days of treatment [48].

Sample collection, storage, handling and DNA extraction techniques all also have the potential to impact on subsequent sequencing results. For example, multiple freeze–thaw cycles have been demonstrated to affect the results of microbiota analysis in respiratory samples [49]. Furthermore, different sequencing platforms can also produce different profiles [50].

There is no universally standardised protocol for the extraction of DNA from respiratory samples, and hence methods are often inconsistent between study groups. One obvious inconsistency is the use of propidium monoazide (PMA), a chemical compound that binds DNA in cells with damaged membranes and hence allows exclusion of non-viable DNA from sequencing. Excluding non-viable DNA has been suggested to be important for accurately identifying which members of the community are active at times of exacerbation and helps to avoid overestimation of viable microorganisms following treatment with antibiotics, but it is not utilised by all groups [51, 52]. There are concerns that PMA may incompletely penetrate sputum, hence only identifying a portion of non-viable cells. PMA is also known to stain viable cells of some species and stain dead cells in others [53]. In CF exacerbations, PMA treatment was not found to significantly alter the community as a whole, and only changes in low abundance 'satellite' taxa were apparent [51].

Overall, there is certainly evidence that acute antibiotic administration alters the respiratory microbiota; however, in the absence of prospective controlled trials, it is difficult to interpret these results given the confounders mentioned above. Indeed there have been calls for future clinical trials in CF to include biobanking of samples to allow a more rigorous scrutiny of the effect of antibiotic agents on the microbiome [54].

7. Community changes associated with chronic suppressive antibiotics

Inhaled antibiotics such as colistimethate (COL), tobramycin (TOB), aztreonam (AZLI) and levofloxacin (LIS) preparations are all licenced in the UK for the treatment of chronic *P. aeruginosa* infections and have, to varying degrees, demonstrated improvements in lung function and exacerbation rates as well as sputum density of *P. aeruginosa* [55–58]. However, despite the near ubiquitous use of these inhaled anti-pseudomonals in the chronic *P. aeruginosa* treatment in CF, the effect of these treatments on the microbiome remains poorly defined. Furthermore, many patients receive chronic macrolide therapy over many years, at least in part for its immunomodulatory effects, yet similarly little is known about the effects of this persistent selective pressure on the microbiota. When considering inhaled antibiotics, there is contrasting evidence as to their influence on the CF microbiome. For example, Kramer et al. [59] did not find any correlation between bacterial community structure and inhaled antibiotic treatments, although it is unclear which agents patients were using in that study. More recently Acosta et al. [24] utilised a prospectively collected Canadian sputum biobank primarily to investigate changes in CF cohort microbiota over time but also assessed whether different long-term antibiotics were associated with distinct microbiota. Eighty-two samples from 42 patients were sequenced, and those receiving long-term tobramycin and colistimethate harboured significantly different respiratory communities compared to those who were not, but interestingly no differences were seen in people receiving AZLI. The authors also assessed the impact of long-term oral azithromycin and nebulised dornase, but these agents were not associated with any differences. Perhaps intrigued by the failure of AZLI to be associated with microbiomic differences given its proven clinical benefits, the same group investigated its effects in more detail. In the only published study focussing on the microbiomic outcomes of a specific inhaled antibiotic, Heirali et al. [54] utilised the same Canadian biobank and sequenced 80 samples from 24 patients naive to AZLI and 82 samples from the same patients following initiation of AZLI. Overall no differences were observed in alpha or beta diversity measures, but at the OTU level, significantly lower relative abundances of *Prevotella* were seen following AZLI initiation. The authors then subclassified patients into AZLI 'responders' and 'non-responders' based on clinical outcomes and found 'non-responders' to have lower abundance of *Pseudomonas* and higher abundance of *Staphylococcus*. This novel approach raises the prospect of signatures in an individual's microbiota acting as a biomarker for response to antibiotics and may represent an important step in the march towards personalised precision medicine in CF. Further studies are required to explore the potential for an individual's microbiota to guide treatment.

8. Community changes associated with CFTR modulators

In the last 5 years, treatments targeted towards correcting the underlying defect in CF have become available. Ivacaftor, a cystic fibrosis transmembrane conductance regulator (CFTR) potentiator, is licenced specifically for the treatment of people with a G551D mutation and a number of other rare gating mutations, which together account for approximately 5–10% of the CF population in the UK [60]. In this subset of the CF population, ivacaftor use has been associated with improvements in lung function, reductions in exacerbations, reductions in sweat chloride, improved weight gain and improved quality of life [61, 62]. The restoration of CFTR activity by ivacaftor and the associated clinical benefits, in particular improved lung function and reductions in exacerbation, has inevitably raised questions as to whether ivacaftor has an antimicrobial effect.

Theoretically, ivacaftor could have an antimicrobial effect in a number of ways. Firstly, the restoration of CFTR activity should result in a rehydrated airway surface layer, and this in turn will allow the mucociliary escalator to function physiologically. The improved clearance of airway secretions would then result in the elimination of bacteria. Secondly, the restoration of CFTR activity could result in a dramatic change in the local pulmonary microenvironment, turning a previously favourable environmental niche into an inhospitable one for resident microbiota. There is evidence to support a similar effect in the GI tract, where CFTR modulation with ivacaftor was associated with improved proximal small intestinal pH, likely secondary to improved bicarbonate secretion [63]. Thirdly, a direct bactericidal effect of ivacaftor itself has been postulated given that its chemical structure contains a quinolone ring and many quinolone derivatives have antimicrobial properties [64]. This theory is supported by evidence that ivacaftor exerted in vitro antibacterial effects on clinical respiratory isolates of *S. aureus* (MSSA and MRSA) and *Streptococcus pneumoniae* [65, 66]. However, these studies found very little activity against Gram-negative organisms, which is uncharacteristic of a quinolone-based antibiotic [65]. Interestingly, the authors of the same study noted synergism of ivacaftor with antibiotics commonly used in CF, and this was recently supported by Payne et al., who again found that ivacaftor had activity against *Streptococcus* spp. and *S. aureus* and that the effect was potentiated in the presence of tobramycin. Again there was no evidence of direct antibacterial activity against *P. aeruginosa* [67].

Interest has since focussed on clinical microbiological outcomes of patients commenced on ivacaftor therapy in an effort to investigate differences post-treatment initiation. Interestingly, despite ivacaftor appearing to have no innate activity against *P. aeruginosa,* a number of studies have reported reductions in counts and density post initiation, perhaps suggesting that quinolone activity is not the only mechanism at play [68, 69].

In contrast to the relative lack of focus on inhaled antibiotics, a number of studies have investigated the effects of ivacaftor on the respiratory microbiome. Peleg et al. [70] conducted the only placebo-controlled trial in this field when they performed a double-blind, placebo-controlled, cross-over study of 28-day ivacaftor treatment. Sputum was collected at the start and end of each 28-day treatment period, and 16S rRNA sequencing with qPCR correlation was subsequently performed. No significant differences were observed for either total bacterial load or *P. aeruginosa* load following ivacaftor therapy, and no significant difference in the microbiota composition (based on 16S rRNA microbiome analysis) was observed between the placebo and treatment samples. However, the authors noted that when they adjusted for consistent or changing antibiotic exposure in the 28-day study period, ivacaftor was associated with a significant reduction in *P. aeruginosa* load. That is to say, changes in the microbiota induced by acute changes in antibiotic administration during the 28-day treatment periods may have masked the effect induced by ivacaftor.

In longer-term observational studies, a number of changes have been observed. Bernarde et al. [71] noted no significant changes in bacteria load and also no significant changes in overall community composition at 1 year following ivacaftor initiation. However, individual taxa were observed to change in that the relative abundance of *Streptococcus mitis* group was significantly diminished and a *Porphyromonas* OTU was significantly increased. Elsewhere, in perhaps the most comprehensive study of microbiological outcomes following ivacaftor initiation, Hisert et al. [72] found marked reductions in *P. aeruginosa* sputum densities using conventional culture and also reduced sputum inflammatory markers in regular follow-up throughout the first 2 years of ivacaftor use. These findings were mirrored in the 16S rRNA-based analysis, where decreases in mean *P. aeruginosa* relative abundance and subsequent increases in diversity measures were observed. However, no patient eradicated *P. aeruginosa*, and after 12 months of treatment, relative abundance, sputum counts and inflammatory markers began to increase again. The authors interpreted these findings to suggest that *P. aeruginosa* may adapt to a CFTR-restored environment and this clearly has implications for the need for ongoing anti-infective chemotherapy in CF.

9. Nontuberculous mycobacteria

Nontuberculous mycobacteria (NTM) are identified in approximately 10% of CF patients, but only a small proportion will go on to develop NTM pulmonary disease (NTM-PD) warranting treatment. First and foremost, the management of CF pulmonary disease should be optimised, including antibiotic therapy targeted to the individual's usual airway bacteria, prior to considering treatment for NTM-PD. Those who fulfil criteria for NTM lung disease may not necessarily require treatment and could be monitored expectantly if symptoms and radiographic findings are minimal or stable over a period of surveillance. However, the presence of *Mycobacterium abscessus* complex (MABSC), deteriorating lung function, worsening radiology and/or anticipated lung transplant should prompt NTM therapy initiation (**Table 2**). For CF patients with *Mycobacterium avium* complex (MAC), recommended treatment includes triple antibiotic therapy with a macrolide, rifampin and ethambutol. Azithromycin is generally the preferred macrolide of choice in CF as it is better tolerated and has fewer drug–drug interactions. An initial course of injectable amikacin or streptomycin should be considered in the presence of (i) acid-fast bacillus smear-positive respiratory tract samples, (ii) radiological evidence of lung cavitation or severe infection and (iii) systemic signs of illness. MABSC treatment is more complicated and requires an induction phase (oral macrolide and two IV agents including amikacin with one or more additional intravenous antibiotics including tigecycline, imipenem, cefoxitin) for 3 to 12 weeks as well as a maintenance phase (nebulised amikacin and a macrolide with two to three oral antibiotics including minocycline, clofazimine, moxifloxacin, linezolid). Baseline and interval testing for drug toxicity is essential. The treatment duration for both MAC and MABSC is extended 1-year post-culture conversion. However, in patients who do not achieve culture negative status but tolerate therapy, ongoing treatment for mycobacterial suppression and prevention of disease progression can be considered. There are no randomised controlled trials of MABSC therapy in the general population or in CF; however, there is MABSC treatment outcome data in non-CF populations from several clinical studies [74]. In a study of 57 non-CF

Clinical (both required)

1. Pulmonary symptoms with nodular or cavitary opacities on chest radiograph or a high-resolution CT scan that shows multifocal bronchiectasis with multiple small nodules
2. Appropriate exclusion of other diagnoses.

Microbiologic (one of the following required)

- Positive culture results from at least two expectorated sputum samples. If the results from samples are non-diagnostic, consider repeat sputum acid-fast bacillus (AFB) smears and cultures.
- Positive culture results from at least one bronchial wash or lavage.
- Transbronchial or other lung biopsy with mycobacterial histopathological features (granulomatous inflammation or AFB) and positive culture for NTM or biopsy showing mycobacterial histopathological features (granulomatous inflammation or AFB) and one or more sputum or bronchial washings that are culture positive for NTM.
- Expert consultation should be obtained when either infrequently encountered NTM or those usually representing environmental contamination are recovered.
- Patients who are suspected of having NTM-PD but who do not meet the diagnostic criteria should be followed up until the diagnosis is firmly established or excluded.
- Making the diagnosis of NTM-PD does not, per se, necessitate the institution of therapy, which is a decision based on potential risks and benefits of therapy for individual patients.

Table 2.
ATS/IDSA clinical and microbiologic criteria for diagnosing nontuberculous mycobacterial pulmonary disease (NTM-PD) [73].

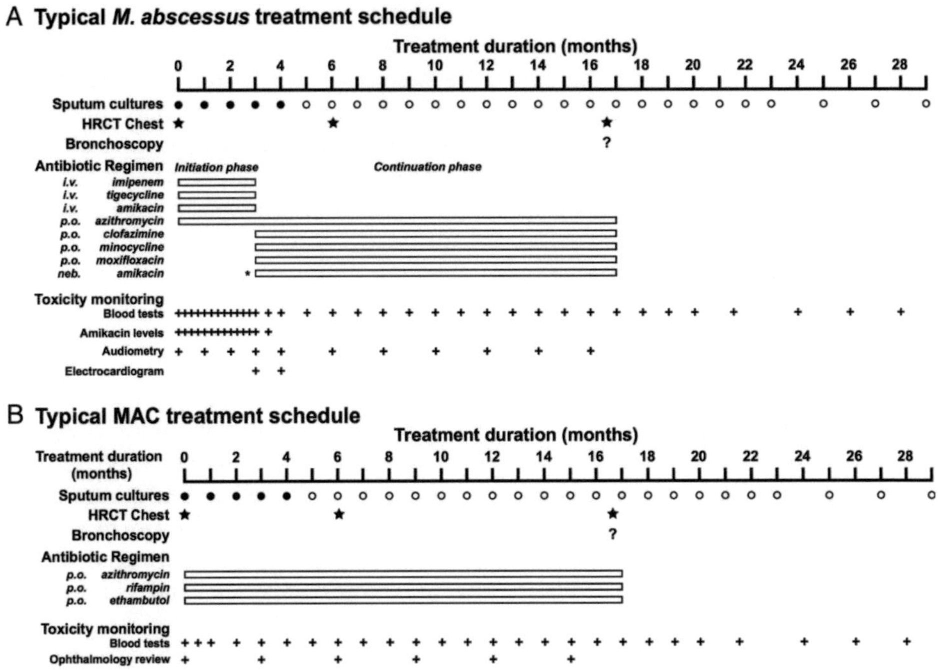

Figure 2.
Typical treatment schedules for individuals with CF with Mycobacterium abscessus *or MAC pulmonary disease [74].*

subjects that compared *M. abscessus* ssp. *massiliense* and ssp. *abscessus* infections and treatment outcomes, all individuals were treated with clarithromycin-containing regimen in combination with an initial 4-week course of cefoxitin and amikacin, was given to 57 patients (24 with *M. abscessus* and 33 with *M. massiliense*) for more than 12 months. The proportion of patients with sputum conversion and maintenance of negative sputum cultures was higher in patients with *M. massiliense* infection (88%) than in those with *M. abscessus* infection (25%; $p < 0.001$). Inducible resistance to clarithromycin (minimal inhibitory concentrations ≥ 32 μg/ml) was found in all tested *M. abscessus* isolates (n = 19), but in none of the *M. massiliense* isolates (n = 28) [75].

Inhaled liposomal amikacin for maintenance treatment has also drawn interest. In a randomised placebo-controlled trial, CF subjects with NTM lung disease refractory to standard therapy were assigned to 590 mg OD inhaled liposomal amikacin or placebo, in addition to their standard CF treatments and ongoing NTM therapy [76]. The group of 90 patients was stratified based on MAC (64%) and MABSC (36%) [77]. At the end of the 6-month treatment period, there was a statistically significant increase in culture negativity overall and for the MAC group.

Reported NTM prevalence in CF ranges from 3 [78] to 23% [79]. The majority (95%) of NTM isolated from CF patients are *Mycobacterium avium* complex (MAC) (*M. avium-intracellulare* and four *M. avium* subspecies) and *M. abscessus* complex (MABSC) (subspecies abscessus, massiliense, and bolletii) [80, 81]. Bryant et al. [82] reported the largest outbreak occurred in Cambridge, England, where 11 of 31 patients with MABSC had a shared strain of *M. abscessus* subsp. *massiliense* with similar antibiotic resistance patterns by whole genome sequencing despite a lack of exposure to the same antibiotics, raising the possibility of cross infection amongst the CF cohort albeit conventional cross infection measures (**Figure 2**).

MABSC has been demonstrated to accelerate lung function decline in CF patients compared to uninfected CF controls [83, 84]. In CF, a common measure of lung disease severity is percent-predicted forced expiratory volume in 1 second (FEV1), with lower values indicating more severe lung disease. Qvist et al. showed that MABSC had a greater rate of FEV1% predicted decline than other organisms, including *Pseudomonas aeruginosa* and *Burkholderia cepacia* [84]. However, no lung function decline was noted in patients growing MAC [83]. Likewise, a large study found no significant effect of NTM infection on lung function decline, although analyses were not based on different NTM subtypes [80]. A diagnosis of NTM pulmonary disease must meet both clinical and microbiologic criteria as outlined by ATS guidelines, with exclusion of other aetiologies [73].

Individuals who are NTM culture positive but who do not meet ATS criteria for disease should be monitored closely [74]. Patients with CF meeting criteria for NTM-PD should be considered for therapy; however, treatment decisions should be individualised [74, 85]. It may be reasonable to monitor individuals with mild CF lung disease, MAC lung disease with mild symptoms and radiographic changes or a high possibility of drug intolerance or drug interactions [85]. However, CF patients with MABSC and/or severe CF lung disease should generally be treated in the absence of contraindications [85].

10. Fungal lung disease in CF

Clinical manifestations of respiratory fungal diseases in adult CF patients are very heterogeneous, ranging from asymptomatic colonisation to chronic infections, allergic disorders or invasive diseases in immunosuppressed CF patients following lung transplantation.

Aspergillus spp. are amongst the most widespread filamentous fungi in the environment, especially in areas with high humidity [86]. In CF patients, the most frequently isolated species is *Aspergillus fumigatus*, accounting for 67–73% of *Aspergillus*-positive sputum cultures [87]. Isolation of other species such as *A. flavus*, *A. niger* and *A. terreus* is less frequent but not rare (4, 4 and 2% of *Aspergillus*-positive sputum cultures, respectively) [87]. Notably, the prevalence of isolation of *Aspergillus* spp. from sputum cultures in CF patients increases with age, possibly reaching 46–78% in adult CF patients, although with important inter-region and inter-centre variability [88–90]. However, knowledge of the prevalence of *Aspergillus* spp. isolation from sputum does not automatically allow to infer the prevalence of the various *Aspergillus*-related manifestations in CF patients, which range from asymptomatic colonisation to invasive diseases, especially in patients post-lung transplantation.

Allergic bronchopulmonary aspergillosis (ABPA) refers to a complex hypersensitivity reaction which often occurs in patients affected by CF or asthma. ABPA is beyond the scope of discussion in this chapter.

In CF patients, the disease-related progressive damage of the lungs may favour the development of chronic *Aspergillus* infection, commonly defined as '*Aspergillus* bronchitis', although aspergilloma(s) might also develop in some cases, especially in pre-existing cavities or bronchiectasis [91–93]. *Aspergillus* bronchitis has an estimated prevalence of ~2–8% in CF patients and may be suspected in the case of pulmonary exacerbation unresponsive to antibacterial treatment [94, 95]. As per Baxter et al.'s [96] classification, diagnosis of *Aspergillus* bronchitis can be made in the presence of a positive sputum galactomannan, high levels of *Aspergillus*-specific IgG and negative total and *Aspergillus*-specific IgE. Since *Aspergillus* bronchitis does reflect infection and not an immune-mediated response as in ABPA, corticosteroids are not the cornerstone of treatment. Treatment with azole derivatives is the current standard of care, although the overall duration of treatment is still not clearly defined [97]. Invasive aspergillosis is described as the infection progresses across tissues and invades the vessels, with subsequent necrosis [96]. Usually, invasive aspergillosis is observed in severely immunocompromised non-CF populations, such as haematology patients with prolonged neutropenia and patients receiving high dosages of corticosteroids or other immunosuppressive agents. Clinical symptoms usually include fever, chest pain, shortness of breath and/or cough [96]. Haemoptysis and pneumothorax might also develop in some cases [98, 99]. Invasive aspergillosis is rarely seen in patients affected by CF. However, it could develop in end-stage CF patient and in immunosuppressed CF patients following lung transplantation, frequently in the form of *Aspergillus* tracheobronchitis, occurring mainly in the first 3 months after transplants and associated with increased mortality (39%) [100, 101]. Frequent symptoms of *Aspergillus* tracheobronchitis are severe dyspnoea, cough and wheezing [97]. The histopathological examination may show different features: (1) obstructive bronchial aspergillosis; (2) ulcerative tracheobronchitis (characterised by the invasion of the tracheobronchial mucosa and cartilage); and (3) pseudomembranous tracheobronchitis (characterised by inflammation and invasion of the tracheobronchial tree). Invasive aspergillosis is usually treated with systemic azole therapy (possibly associated with nebulised amphotericin B in some cases of tracheobronchitis) [97]. The US guidelines recommend a minimum of 6 to 12 weeks of therapy for patients with invasive pulmonary aspergillosis and at least 3 months in the case of *Aspergillus* tracheobronchitis [97].

11. Conclusion

The pulmonary microbiome of people with CF diverging significantly from that of the healthy individuals has been the focus of much research in the last 5 years often producing more questions than answers. As the disease progresses, community structure becomes progressively less diverse, most likely as a consequence of long-term aggressive antibiotic therapy. The impact of acute antibiotic therapy, antifungal treatments and CFTR modulators are less well defined, and prospective clinical trials with sputum biobanking are needed to answer these questions.

Author details

Freddy J. Frost, Dilip Nazareth and Dennis Wat*
Liverpool Heart and Chest Hospital, Liverpool, UK

*Address all correspondence to: dennis.wat@lhch.nhs.uk

References

[1] Round JL, Mazmanian SK. The gut microbiota shapes intestinal immune responses during health and disease. Nature Reviews. Immunology. 2009;**9**(5):313-323

[2] Larsbrink J et al. A discrete genetic locus confers xyloglucan metabolism in select human gut bacteroidetes. Nature. 2014;**506**(7489):498-502

[3] Cebra JJ. Influences of microbiota on intestinal immune system development. The American Journal of Clinical Nutrition. 1999;**69**(5):1046S-1051S

[4] Ley RE et al. Microbial ecology: Human gut microbes associated with obesity. Nature. 2006;**444**(7122):1022-1023

[5] Brunkwall L, Orho-Melander M. The gut microbiome as a target for prevention and treatment of hyperglycaemia in type 2 diabetes: From current human evidence to future possibilities. Diabetologia. 2017;**60**(6):943-951

[6] Lane ER, Zisman TL, Suskind DL. The microbiota in inflammatory bowel disease: Current and therapeutic insights. Journal of Inflammation Research. 2017;**10**:63-73

[7] Cox MJ et al. Airway microbiota and pathogen abundance in age-stratified cystic fibrosis patients. PLoS One. 2010;**5**(6):e11044

[8] Dickson RP et al. The microbiome and the respiratory tract. Annual Review of Physiology. 2016;**78**:481-504

[9] Hilty M et al. Disordered microbial communities in asthmatic airways. PLoS One. 2010;**5**(1):e8578

[10] Cox MJ, Cookson WO, Moffatt MF. Sequencing the human microbiome in health and disease. Human Molecular Genetics. 2013;**22**(R1):R88-R94

[11] Dickson RP, Huffnagle GB. The lung microbiome: New principles for respiratory bacteriology in health and disease. PLoS Pathogens. 2015;**11**(7):e1004923

[12] Prevaes SM et al. Concordance between upper and lower airway microbiota in infants with cystic fibrosis. The European Respiratory Journal. 2017;**49**(3):1602235

[13] Prevaes SM et al. Development of the nasopharyngeal microbiota in infants with cystic fibrosis. American Journal of Respiratory and Critical Care Medicine. 2016;**193**(5):504-515

[14] Mika M et al. The nasal microbiota in infants with cystic fibrosis in the first year of life: A prospective cohort study. The Lancet Respiratory Medicine. 2016;**4**(8):627-635

[15] Boutin S et al. Comparison of oropharyngeal microbiota from children with asthma and cystic fibrosis. Mediators of Inflammation. 2017;**2017**:5047403

[16] Boutin S et al. Comparison of microbiomes from different niches of upper and lower airways in children and adolescents with cystic fibrosis. PLoS One. 2015;**10**(1):e0116029

[17] Muhlebach MS et al. Initial acquisition and succession of the cystic fibrosis lung microbiome is associated with disease progression in infants and preschool children. PLoS Pathogens. 2018;**14**(1):e1006798

[18] Coburn B et al. Lung microbiota across age and disease stage in cystic fibrosis. Scientific Reports. 2015;**5**:10241

[19] Zhao J et al. Decade-long bacterial community dynamics in cystic fibrosis airways. Proceedings of the National Academy of Sciences of the United States of America. 2012;**109**(15):5809-5814

[20] Fodor AA et al. The adult cystic fibrosis airway microbiota is stable over time and infection type, and highly resilient to antibiotic treatment of exacerbations. PLoS One. 2012;**7**(9):e45001

[21] Stokell JR et al. Analysis of changes in diversity and abundance of the microbial community in a cystic fibrosis patient over a multiyear period. Journal of Clinical Microbiology. 2015;**53**(1):237-247

[22] Whelan FJ et al. Longitudinal sampling of the lung microbiota in individuals with cystic fibrosis. PLoS One. 2017;**12**(3):e0172811

[23] Whelan FJ, Surette MG. Clinical insights into pulmonary exacerbations in cystic fibrosis from the microbiome. What are we missing? Annals of the American Thoracic Society. 2015;**12**(Suppl 2):S207-S211

[24] Acosta N et al. The evolving cystic fibrosis microbiome: A comparative cohort study spanning sixteen years. Annals of the American Thoracic Society. 2017;**14**(8):1288-1297

[25] VanDevanter DR, LiPuma JJ. Microbial diversity in the cystic fibrosis airways: Where is thy sting? Future Microbiology. 2012;**7**(7):801-803

[26] Bacci G, Mengoni A, Fiscarelli E, et al. A different microbiome gene repertoire in the airways of cystic fibrosis patients with severe lung disease. International Journal of Molecular Sciences. 2017;**18**(8):1654. Published 29 July 2017. DOI: 10.3390/ijms18081654

[27] Bacci G et al. Pyrosequencing unveils cystic fibrosis lung microbiome differences associated with a severe lung function decline. PLoS One. 2016;**11**(6):e0156807

[28] Paganin P et al. Changes in cystic fibrosis airway microbial community associated with a severe decline in lung function. PLoS One. 2015;**10**(4):e0124348

[29] Zhao J, Murray S, Lipuma JJ. Modeling the impact of antibiotic exposure on human microbiota. Scientific Reports. 2014;**4**:4345

[30] Caverly LJ et al. Episodic oral antibiotic use in CF: Discordance between the electronic medical record and self-report. Journal of Cystic Fibrosis. 2016;**15**(5):630-633

[31] Pittman JE et al. Association of Antibiotics, airway microbiome, and inflammation in infants with cystic fibrosis. Annals of the American Thoracic Society. 2017;**14**(10):1548-1555

[32] Britto MT et al. Impact of recent pulmonary exacerbations on quality of life in patients with cystic fibrosis. Chest. 2002;**121**(1):64-72

[33] Sanders DB et al. Pulmonary exacerbations are associated with subsequent FEV1 decline in both adults and children with cystic fibrosis. Pediatric Pulmonology. 2011;**46**(4):393-400

[34] Price KE et al. Unique microbial communities persist in individual cystic fibrosis patients throughout a clinical exacerbation. Microbiome. 2013;**1**(1):27

[35] Cuthbertson L, Rogers G, Walker A, et al. Respiratory microbiota resistance and resilience to pulmonary exacerbation and subsequent antimicrobial intervention. The ISME Journal. 2016;**10**(5):1081-1091

[36] Filkins LM et al. Prevalence of streptococci and increased polymicrobial diversity associated with cystic fibrosis patient stability. Journal of Bacteriology. 2012;**194**(17):4709-4717

[37] Li J et al. Data mining of lung microbiota in cystic fibrosis patients. PLoS One. 2016;**11**(10):e0164510

[38] Carmody LA et al. The daily dynamics of cystic fibrosis airway microbiota during clinical stability and at exacerbation. Microbiome. 2015;**3**:12

[39] Bafadhel M et al. Acute exacerbations of chronic obstructive pulmonary disease: Identification of biologic clusters and their biomarkers. American Journal of Respiratory and Critical Care Medicine. 2011;**184**(6):662-671

[40] Twomey KB et al. Microbiota and metabolite profiling reveal specific alterations in bacterial community structure and environment in the cystic fibrosis airway during exacerbation. PLoS One. 2013;**8**(12):e82432

[41] Quinn RA et al. Ecological networking of cystic fibrosis lung infections. NPJ Biofilms Microbiomes. 2016;**2**:4

[42] Carmody LA et al. Changes in cystic fibrosis airway microbiota at pulmonary exacerbation. Annals of the American Thoracic Society. 2013;**10**(3):179-187

[43] Waite RD, Qureshi MR, Whiley RA. Modulation of behaviour and virulence of a high alginate expressing *Pseudomonas aeruginosa* strain from cystic fibrosis by oral commensal bacterium *Streptococcus anginosus*. PLoS One. 2017;**12**(3):e0173741

[44] Scoffield JA et al. A commensal streptococcus hijacks a *Pseudomonas aeruginosa* exopolysaccharide to promote biofilm formation. PLoS Pathogens. 2017;**13**(4):e1006300

[45] Daniels TW et al. Impact of antibiotic treatment for pulmonary exacerbations on bacterial diversity in cystic fibrosis. Journal of Cystic Fibrosis. 2013;**12**(1):22-28

[46] Zemanick ET et al. Inflammation and airway microbiota during cystic fibrosis pulmonary exacerbations. PLoS One. 2013;**8**(4):e62917

[47] Alton EWFW, Armstrong DK, Ashby D, et al. on behalf of the UK Cystic Fibrosis Gene Therapy Consortium. A Randomised, Double-Blind, Placebo-Controlled Trial of Repeated Nebulisation of Non-Viral Cystic Fibrosis Transmembrane Conductance Regulator (CFTR) Gene Therapy in Patients with Cystic Fibrosis. Southampton (UK): NIHR Journals Library (Efficacy and Mechanism Evaluation, No. 3.5.); July 2016

[48] Smith DJ et al. Pyrosequencing reveals transient cystic fibrosis lung microbiome changes with intravenous antibiotics. The European Respiratory Journal. 2014;**44**(4):922-930

[49] Cuthbertson L et al. Implications of multiple freeze-thawing on respiratory samples for culture-independent analyses. Journal of Cystic Fibrosis. 2015;**14**(4):464-467

[50] Hahn A et al. Different next generation sequencing platforms produce different microbial profiles and diversity in cystic fibrosis sputum. Journal of Microbiological Methods. 2016;**130**:95-99

[51] Nguyen LD et al. Effects of propidium monoazide (PMA) treatment on mycobiome and bacteriome analysis of cystic fibrosis airways during exacerbation. PLoS One. 2016;**11**(12):e0168860

[52] Rogers GB et al. Reducing bias in bacterial community analysis of

lower respiratory infections. The ISME Journal. 2013;**7**(4):697-706

[53] Emerson JB et al. Schrodinger's microbes: Tools for distinguishing the living from the dead in microbial ecosystems. Microbiome. 2017;**5**(1):86

[54] Heirali AA et al. The effects of inhaled aztreonam on the cystic fibrosis lung microbiome. Microbiome. 2017;**5**(1):51

[55] Assael BM et al. Inhaled aztreonam lysine vs. inhaled tobramycin in cystic fibrosis: A comparative efficacy trial. Journal of Cystic Fibrosis. 2013;**12**(2):130-140

[56] Elborn JS, Flume PA, Cohen F, et al. Safety and efficacy of prolonged levofloxacin inhalation solution (APT-1026) treatment for cystic fibrosis and chronic *Pseudomonas aeruginosa* airway infection. Journal of Cystic Fibrosis. 2016;**15**:634-640

[57] Conole D, Keating GM. Colistimethate sodium dry powder for inhalation: A review of its use in the treatment of chronic *Pseudomonas aeruginosa* infection in patients with cystic fibrosis. Drugs. 2014;**74**(3):377-387

[58] Hodson ME, Gallagher CG. New clinical evidence from the European tobramycin trial in cystic fibrosis. Journal of Cystic Fibrosis. 2002;**1**(Suppl 2):199-202

[59] Kramer R et al. High individuality of respiratory bacterial communities in a large cohort of adult cystic fibrosis patients under continuous antibiotic treatment. PLoS One. 2015;**10**(2):e0117436

[60] Sermet-Gaudelus I. Ivacaftor treatment in patients with cystic fibrosis and the G551D-CFTR mutation. European Respiratory Review. 2013;**22**(127):66-71

[61] Ramsey BW et al. A CFTR potentiator in patients with cystic fibrosis and the G551D mutation. The New England Journal of Medicine. 2011;**365**(18):1663-1672

[62] Sawicki GS et al. Sustained benefit from ivacaftor demonstrated by combining clinical trial and cystic fibrosis patient registry data. American Journal of Respiratory and Critical Care Medicine. 2015;**192**(7):836-842

[63] Gelfond D et al. Impact of CFTR modulation on intestinal pH, motility, and clinical outcomes in patients with cystic fibrosis and the G551D mutation. Clinical and Translational Gastroenterology. 2017;**8**(3):e81

[64] Aldred KJ, Kerns RJ, Osheroff N. Mechanism of quinolone action and resistance. Biochemistry. 2014;**53**(10):1565-1574

[65] Reznikov LR et al. Antibacterial properties of the CFTR potentiator ivacaftor. Journal of Cystic Fibrosis. 2014;**13**(5):515-519

[66] Thakare R et al. Repurposing ivacaftor for treatment of *Staphylococcus aureus* infections. International Journal of Antimicrobial Agents. 2017;**50**(3):389-392

[67] Payne JE et al. Activity of innate antimicrobial peptides and ivacaftor against clinical cystic fibrosis respiratory pathogens. International Journal of Antimicrobial Agents. 2017;**50**(3):427-435

[68] Millar BC et al. *Pseudomonas aeruginosa* in cystic fibrosis patients with c.1652GA (G551D)-CFTR treated with ivacaftor-changes in microbiological parameters. Journal of Clinical Pharmacy and Therapeutics. 2018;**43**(1):92-100

[69] Heltshe SL et al. *Pseudomonas aeruginosa* in cystic fibrosis patients

with G551D-CFTR treated with ivacaftor. Clinical Infectious Diseases. 2015;**60**(5):703-712

[70] Peleg AY et al. Antibiotic exposure and interpersonal variance mask the effect of ivacaftor on respiratory microbiota composition. Journal of Cystic Fibrosis. 2018;**17**(1):50-56

[71] Bernarde C et al. Impact of the CFTR-potentiator ivacaftor on airway microbiota in cystic fibrosis patients carrying a G551D mutation. PLoS One. 2015;**10**(4):e0124124

[72] Hisert KB et al. Restoring cystic fibrosis transmembrane conductance regulator function reduces airway bacteria and inflammation in people with cystic fibrosis and chronic lung infections. American Journal of Respiratory and Critical Care Medicine. 2017;**195**(12):1617-1628

[73] Griffith DE, Aksamit T, Brown-Elliott BA, Catanzaro A, Daley C, Gordin F, et al. An official ATS/IDSA statement: Diagnosis, treatment, and prevention of nontuberculous mycobacterial diseases. American Journal of Respiratory and Critical Care Medicine. 2007;**175**(4):367-416

[74] Floto RA, Olivier KN, Saiman L, Daley CL, Herrmann JL, Nick JA, et al. US Cystic Fibrosis Foundation and European cystic fibrosis society consensus recommendations for the management of non-tuberculous mycobacteria in individuals with cystic fibrosis. Thorax. 2016;**71**(Suppl 1):i1-i22

[75] Koh WJ, Jeon K, Lee NY, Kim BJ, Kook YH, Lee SH, et al. Clinical significance of differentiation of *Mycobacterium massiliense* from *Mycobacterium abscessus*. American Journal of Respiratory and Critical Care Medicine. 2011;**183**(3):405-410

[76] Jeon K, Kwon OJ, Lee NY, Kim BJ, Kook YH, Lee SH, et al. Antibiotic treatment of *Mycobacterium abscessus* lung disease: A retrospective analysis of 65 patients. American Journal of Respiratory and Critical Care Medicine. 2009;**180**(9):896-902

[77] Biller JA, Eagle G, McInnis JP et al. Efficacy of Liposomal Amikacin (lai) in achieving nontuberculous mycobacteria (ntm) culture negativity in patients whose lung function is refractory to guideline based therapy. AJRCCM. 2015. Poster Presentation.

[78] Viviani L, Harrison MJ, Zolin A, Haworth CS, Floto RA. Epidemiology of nontuberculous mycobacteria (NTM) amongst individuals with cystic fibrosis (CF). Journal of Cystic Fibrosis. 2016;**15**(5):619-623

[79] Levy I, Grisaru-Soen G, Lerner-Geva L, et al. Multicenter cross-sectional study of nontuberculous mycobacterial infections among cystic fibrosis patients Israel. Emerging Infectious Diseases. 2008;**14**:378-384

[80] Olivier KN, Weber DJ, Wallace RJ Jr, et al. Nontuberculous mycobacteria. I: Multicenter prevalence study in cystic fibrosis. American Journal of Respiratory and Critical Care Medicine. 2003;**167**:828-834

[81] Pierre-AudigierC FA, Sermet-Gaudelus I, et al. Age-related prevalence and distribution of nontuberculous mycobacterial species among patients with cystic fibrosis. Journal of Clinical Microbiology. 2005;**43**:3467-3470

[82] Bryant JM, Grogono DM, Greaves D, Foweraker J, Roddick I, Inns T, et al. Whole-genome sequencing to identify transmission of *Mycobacterium abscessus* between patients with cystic fibrosis: A retrospective cohort study. Lancet. 2013;**381**(9877):1551-1560

[83] Esther CR Jr, Henry MM, Molina PL, Leigh MW. Nontuberculous

mycobacterial infection in young children with cystic fibrosis. Pediatric Pulmonology. 2005;**40**(1):39-44

[84] Qvist T, Taylor-Robinson D, Waldmann E, et al. Comparing the harmful effects of nontuberculous mycobacteria and gram negative bacteria on lung function in patients with cystic fibrosis. Journal of Cystic Fibrosis. 2016;**15**:380-385

[85] Leung JM, Olivier KN. Nontuberculous mycobacteria: The changing epidemiology and treatment challenges in cystic fibrosis. Current Opinion in Pulmonary Medicine. 2013;**19**(6):662-669

[86] Paulussen C, Hallsworth JE, Alvarez-Perez S, et al. Ecology of aspergillosis: Insights into the pathogenic potency of *Aspergillus fumigatus* and some other *Aspergillus* species. Microbial Biotechnology. 2017;**10**:296-322

[87] Mortensen KL, Jensen RH, Johansen HK, et al. *Aspergillus* species and other molds in respiratory samples from patients with cystic fibrosis: A laboratory-based study with focus on *Aspergillus fumigatus* azole resistance. Journal of Clinical Microbiology. 2011;**49**:2243-2251

[88] Bakare N, Rickerts V, Bargon J, Just-Nubling G. Prevalence of *Aspergillus fumigatus* and other fungal species in the sputum of adult patients with cystic fibrosis. Mycoses. 2003;**46**:19-23

[89] Lipuma JJ. The changing microbial epidemiology in cystic fibrosis. Clinical Microbiology Reviews. 2010;**23**:299-323

[90] Valenza G, Tappe D, Turnwald D, et al. Prevalence and antimicrobial susceptibility of microorganisms isolated from sputa of patients with cystic fibrosis. Journal of Cystic Fibrosis. 2008;7:123-127

[91] Amin R, Dupuis A, Aaron SD, Ratjen F. The effect of chronic infection with *Aspergillus fumigatus* on lung function and hospitalization in patients with cystic fibrosis. Chest. 2010;**137**:171-176

[92] Maguire CP, Hayes JP, Hayes M, Masterson J, FitzGerald MX. Three cases of pulmonary aspergilloma in adult patients with cystic fibrosis. Thorax. 1995;**50**:805-806

[93] Pendleton M, Denning DW. Multifocal pulmonary aspergillomas: Case series and review. Annals of the New York Academy of Sciences. 2012;**1272**:58-67

[94] Brandt C, Roehmel J, Rickerts V, Melichar V, Niemann N, Schwarz C. Aspergillus bronchitis in patients with cystic fibrosis. Mycopathologia. 2018;**183**:61-69

[95] Shoseyov D, Brownlee KG, Conway SP, Kerem E. Aspergillus bronchitis in cystic fibrosis. Chest. 2006;**130**:222-226

[96] Baxter CG, Dunn G, Jones AM, Webb K, Gore R, Richardson MD, et al. Novel immunologic classification of aspergillosis in adult cystic fibrosis. The Journal of Allergy and Clinical Immunology. 2013;**132**:560-566

[97] Patterson TF, Thompson GR III, Denning DW, et al. Practice guidelines for the diagnosis and management of aspergillosis: 2016 update by the infectious diseases society of America. Clinical Infectious Diseases. 2016;**63**:e1-e60

[98] Betancourt BY, Garofoli AC, Sandhu JS, Boma N, Sy AM. Pulmonary aspergillosis presenting with recurrent haemoptysis. BML Case Reports. 7 July 2015

[99] Zhang W, Hu Y, Chen L, Gao J, Xie L. Pleural aspergillosis complicated

by recurrent pneumothorax: A case report. Journal of Medical Case Reports. 2010;**4**:180

[100] Fernandez-Ruiz M, Silva JT, San-Juan R, et al. Aspergillus tracheobronchitis: Report of 8 cases and review of the literature. Medicine (Baltimore). 2012;**91**:261-273

[101] Singh N, Husain S. Aspergillus infections after lung transplantation: Clinical differences in type of transplant and implications for management. The Journal of Heart and Lung Transplantation. 2003;**22**:258-266

Chapter 2

Recent Approach in Microbial Pathogen Complications in Patients with Cystic Fibrosis

Salah Abdelbary

Abstract

Cystic fibrosis (CF) is a multisystem genetic disease caused by mutations in the cystic fibrosis transmembrane conductance regulator (CFTR) gene. Microbial infection is the defined characteristics of cystic fibrosis airway disease. This infection is caused by bacteria, fungi, and viruses which increase complications leading to patient death. Additionally, bacterial pathogens including *Haemophilus influenza*, *Staphylococcus aureus*, *Pseudomonas aeruginosa*, nontuberculous mycobacterium (NTM) species, and MRSA are attributed to pulmonary infections. Subsequently, fungal pathogens such as *Candida* sp. and filamentous fungi such as *Aspergillus fumigatus* can also lead to pulmonary infections. On the other hand, *Pseudomonas aeruginosa* is the most common bacterial pathogen leading to complications in CF distal airways disease. Also, *Aspergillus fumigatus* can lead to aspergillus lung diseases including allergic bronchopulmonary aspergillosis and aspergilloma formation. Control of pathogenic microorganisms associated with cystic fibrosis may prevent pulmonary complications and has the potential to improve the prognosis of this life-limiting disease.

Keywords: cystic fibrosis, *Pseudomonas aeruginosa*, *Aspergillus fumigatus*, *Haemophilus influenzae*, MRSA, CFTR, NTM, microbial infection, respiratory diseases

1. Introduction

Cystic fibrosis (CF) is an autosomal recessive disease which basis on a dysfunctional cystic fibrosis transmembrane conductance regulator (CFTR) protein [1]. It is an inherited chronic disease that remains a common cause of morbidity and mortality in affected patients [2]. Also, it is a monogenic autosomal recessive condition affecting approximately 1 in 3000 of the Caucasian population and involves multiple organs, predominantly the lungs, gastrointestinal tract, pancreas, and liver [3].

Mutations in CFTR gene are resulted in defective mucociliary clearance leading to the production of thick and sticky bronchial mucus. This mucus facilitates the entrapment of viruses, bacteria, and fungal spores and acts as a suitable environment for growth of these microorganisms [4]. High morbidity and mortality rates are secondary to recurrent respiratory infections, which, when associated with this obstructive lung disease, lead to respiratory insufficiency [5]. Complex microorganisms and microbial communities can be identified in the distal airways in a variety of respiratory diseases, including CF [6]. Chronic infection is the defined characteristics of CF airway disease. Conditions within the airways of patients living with CF are conducive to colonization by a variety of opportunistic bacterial, viral, and fungal pathogens [7].

Also, bacterial strains that colonize the respiratory tract include *Haemophilus influenzae*, *Staphylococcus aureus*, *Pseudomonas aeruginosa* [8], and *Burkholderia cepacia*; these have been recorded as the main common CF pathogens. Traditionally, *Pseudomonas aeruginosa* has been regarded as the main pathogen in CF, and chronic infections have been linked to disease morbidity and mortality [9]. Little attention has been paid to the role of *Aspergillus* sp. and other filamentous fungi in CF. It has become more apparent, however, that *Aspergillus* sp. may play an important role in chronic lung disease in CF [10]. This chapter discusses the complications of microorganisms in patients with cystic fibrosis, including bacterial, fungal, and viral pathogens and their effects on this disease leading to an increased risk of mortality.

2. Defining causes and history of cystic fibrosis

Cystic fibrosis is a multisystem genetic disease that affects children and young adults [11]. It is caused by mutations in CFTR gene leading to defective or insufficient amounts of functional CFTR protein and causes abnormalities in chloride (Cl), bicarbonate (HCO_3), and sodium (Na) transport across cell membranes with serious consequences on multiple organs. The CF lung disease is characterized by infection and inflammation with eventual bronchiectasis and eventual respiratory failure causing death in over 90% of CF patients [3].

Cystic fibrosis is an autosomal recessively inherited disorder caused by the presence of one of more than 1500 possible mutations in CFTR gene with an occurrence of the clinical disease being 1 in 2500 live births. This mutation leads to the nonfunction or loss of function of CFTR (a cyclic AMP-regulated chloride ion channel) leading to defective chloride ion transport through epithelial cell surfaces [12].

Since its first description in 1938, study of the genetics, pathophysiology, and clinical manifestation of the disease has led to the creation of new therapies and significantly improved quality of life and survival [2].

In CF, the biology and treatment strategies are important to understand for several reasons. Firstly, it is the most common cause of chronic respiratory failure in children and adults. Secondly, CF is a common reason for the dysfunction of pancreatic exocrine in children and adults. Thirdly, the majority also develop pansinusitis. Other potential consequences of CF include diabetes, liver disease, bone disease, and infertility [3].

Advances in research of CF have given a roadmap for the understanding of pathophysiology studies and treatment stages for other severe airway diseases, including chronic obstructive pulmonary disease, non-CF bronchiectasis, and asthma [11].

Survival of individuals with CF has improved significantly over the last half century from a median age of survival of 5 years in the 1970s to 40 years of age as of 2011. There are different reasons for improvement in clinical outcomes including the intense use of antibiotic therapy, advancement in chest physiotherapy, nutritional support, specialized CF units, and introduction of CFTR modulators; however, the majority of CF deaths still occurred in young adult especially in the ages between 21 and 30 years as a consequence of respiratory failure [13]. Recent research also suggests that even asymptomatic genetic carriers for CF may be at risk for subclinical physiological derangements, which can be exacerbated by external stresses and other environmental triggers [14, 15].

3. Microbial complications in patients with cystic fibrosis

Airways of patients with CF are usually infected with various microorganisms. In infected airways of CF patients, microhabitats can develop owing to local differences in the inflammatory reaction between the different focal areas of infection and also as a result of the competing activities of the many co-colonizing microbial populations [16]. Several bacterial strains are major causes of mortality and morbidity and have therefore been studied intensely [12].

3.1 Microbial infection in patients with cystic fibrosis

Chronic infection is a characteristic of CF airway disease. So, conditions in the airways of patients with CF are conducive to forming colonization by different microorganisms such as bacterial, fungal, and viral pathogens. Molecular identification of microorganisms has emphasized and recorded the polymicrobial nature of microbial infections in the CF airway microenvironment. Additionally, changes in airway of CF physiology through the loss of CFTR functionality lead to a variety of immune dysfunctions that permit microbial pathogen colonization and microbial persistence [7].

The prognosis of patients with the hereditary disease CF is substantially dependent on chronic respiratory infection and inflammation [17]. CF lungs are often colonized or infected with a complex microbial species, mainly composed of bacteria, provoking acute and chronic infections [18]. Airway infection accounts for 90% of the morbidity and mortality observed in CF patients. These chronic infections are typically associated with a few bacterial pathogens such as *Pseudomonas aeruginosa*, *Staphylococcus aureus*, and *Burkholderia cepacia* complex [19].

High morbidity and mortality rates in cystic fibrosis patients are secondary to recurrent respiratory infections, which, when associated with this obstructive lung disease, lead to respiratory insufficiency, the main cause of death in these patients [5, 14].

CF lung disease is characterized by progressive colonization of respiratory tract infection by different bacterial strains leading to polymicrobial biofilms. Also, the emergence of nontuberculous mycobacteria (NTM) infections has caused additional challenges to patient management due to their multiresistance nature to antibiotics [20]. These are compounded by the impairment of mucociliary clearance and the inability to mobilize thick secretions within the airways. These result in mucus impaction, microorganism colonization, recurrent infections, persistent inflammation and death from respiratory failure. With improvement in CF prognosis, new challenges emerge, including the management of fungal colonization and infection [1].

3.2 Host-microbe interactions with CF lung infection

Bacterial and fungal infections are hallmarks of CF lung disease. In the era of long-term inhaled antibiotics and increasing CF patient survival, new "emerging" pathogens are detected in CF airways, yet their pathophysiological impact remains largely controversial and incompletely defined. As a consequence to chronic microbial triggers, innate immune cells, particularly neutrophils, are continuously recruited into CF airways where they combat pathogens but also lead to tissue injury through the release of oxidants and proteases. The coordinated interplay between host immune cell activation and pathogens is essential for the outcome of CF lung disease. A better understanding of this phenomena may enhance the survival in CF [21–23].

3.3 Nontuberculous mycobacteria species in patient with cystic fibrosis

NTM are wide environmental microorganisms causing chronic pulmonary infection in lung diseases such as CF. Also, pulmonary disease caused by NTM has a major threat with CF and difficult to diagnose and problematic to treat according to the US Cystic Fibrosis Foundation (CFF) and European Cystic Fibrosis Society (ECFS). Additionally, the most common NTM species identified in CF are the slow-growing *Mycobacterium avium* complex (MAC) including *M. intracellulare*, *M. avium*, and *M. chimaera* and the rapid-growing *M. abscessus* complex (MABSC) including subspecies of *M. a. abscessus*, *M. a. massiliense*, and *M. a. bolletii*. Other less common NTM species include *M. kansasii*, *M. simiae*, and *M. fortuitum* [24].

In addition, there are more than 100 types of NTM, and more are being found every year. The reported prevalence of NTM in CF varies widely from 45 to 40% with *Mycobacterium avium* complex and *Mycobacterium abscessus* complex being the most common [25, 26].

4. Airway colonization process in patients with cystic fibrosis

Colonization of microorganisms in respiratory tract infection within young CF patient includes common pathogens such as *S. aureus* or *H. influenza* then succeeded by *P. aeruginosa* infection in the latter stages of CF.

It is well established that *Pseudomonas aeruginosa* is a frequent and virulent pulmonary pathogen in patients with CF [27]. After a period of intermittent colonization, the organism becomes permanently established and is difficult to eradicate. Most patients with CF become chronically infected with wild-type *P. aeruginosa* strains in early childhood [28]; prevalence increases with age, so that as many as 80% of patients with CF are infected by the time they reach 20 years [27]. During the years following initial colonization, the wild-type strains uniformly mutate into mucoid variants [28]. Conversion to the mucoid phenotype is thought to be driven by the unique CF microenvironment [29–31]. For patients with CF, this conversion results in a significant increase in morbidity and mortality accompanied by a measurable decline in pulmonary function [28]. The mucoid matrix is believed to allow the formation of protected biofilm microcolonies [30, 32] and provide increased resistance to opsonization, phagocytosis, and digestion [33]. Furthermore, resistance to various antibiotics is increased [27, 34].

The potentiality of pathogenic bacterial colony morphotypes in *P. aeruginosa* evolved to a non-swimming phenotype form. So, motility is considered as one of the first steps of *P. aeruginosa* in CF lungs that lead to adaptation steps including biofilm formation and progress to chronic infection. Also, impaired swimming motility seemed to be a candidate to disease marker of *P. aeruginosa* infection development. So far, the pathological changes in the lungs are best studied due to the high mortality rates linked to poorer lung function and recurrent development of infections [18].

Also, the lungs of people with cystic fibrosis are predominantly colonized with *Pseudomonas aeruginosa* using the following mechanism: firstly, reduced mucociliary clearance combined with the malfunction of antibacterial peptides; secondly, impaired defense of the lungs due to low levels of glutathione and nitrous oxide; thirdly, reduced ingestion of bacteria by lung cells; and finally, increased numbers of bacterial receptors [35].

On the other hand, earlier age of infection with *P. aeruginosa* in our population was strongly associated with greater likelihood of severe lung disease later in life, most particularly in those subjects who acquired *P. aeruginosa* before the age 5; the observed association was stronger in females than in males. *P. aeruginosa* infection may be a cause of more severe CF lung disease but may also be a marker of some other processes determining lung function in children with CF [36].

5. Fungal infection in patients with cystic fibrosis

Fungi are generally divided into molds or yeasts with the latter circumferentially shaped with a one-celled thallus. Molds also known as filamentous fungi grow as branching cylindrical hyphae [1]. Aspergillosis is the most well-characterized and well-recognized *Aspergillus* disease in CF, but reported prevalence varies significantly and is likely to be underdiagnosed. Aspergilli are saprophytic, spore-forming, filamentous fungi found ubiquitously in the environment. *A. fumigatus* is the most prevalent species causing human disease and is the species most frequently isolated from the respiratory secretions of CF patients [37].

Yet, the relative contribution of other emerging pathogens, such as *S. maltophilia*, *Aspergillus*, *Candida*, and *Scedosporium* species, remains less precisely defined. *Aspergillus fumigatus* is the only species that is associated with an increased risk for infection with *P. aeruginosa* [9]. *Candida* sp. is found in as many as 70% of patients with CF. The clinical significance of *Candida* in patients with CF is not clearly understood, but most clinicians discount these organisms as not significant [38]. Fungemia caused by *Trichosporon* has been reported in two patients with CF, who were double lung transplant recipients [39]. Some species such as *Exophiala dermatitidis* grow as unicellular fungi (yeast) at human body temperature but in the case of filamentous fungi at room temperature. *Trichosporon* species as of any *Candida* species may produce true mycelium in culture conditions or in host tissues. So, there are variations in isolation and purification of yeast and filamentous fungi. Additionally, some fungal strains are thermotolerant filamentous mycota such as *Aspergillus fumigatus* which are the most common, and others include *Scedosporium* species and *E. dermatitidis* [1]. *A. fumigatus* is frequently detected in respiratory secretions of both adults and children with CF. Once present in the airways, *Aspergillus* can exacerbate lung inflammation, establish infection, and trigger hypersensitivity responses [10].

In patients with CF, complications increased when exposed to *A. fumigatus* spores causing impaired mucociliary clearance and defective innate immune responses leading to accumulation and persistence of fungal spores within the smaller airways. Also, germination of spores leads to the formation of fungal hyphae and release of antigens, phospholipases, proteases, and other virulence factors which damage the airway of epithelial cells and allow a large dose of antigenic factors access to the interstitial and vascular compartments [40].

Also, exotic genera can be found in CF airway secretions, such as *Penicillium*, *Alternaria*, or *Scedosporium*. Some studies provide the first evidence that even healthy airways are not sterile and contain distinct fungi called "pulmonary mycobiome." The kinetics, dynamics, and disease relevance of the pulmonary mycobiome, however, are poorly understood [7]. The majority of yeasts in CF belong to *Candida* species and the most common species such as *Candida albicans* and other yeast strains recorded such as *Candida parapsilosis*, *Candida krusei*, *Candida glabrata*, and *Candida dubliniensis* [1].

6. Viral infection in patients with cystic fibrosis

Progression of CF respiratory disease is influenced by viral infection. Respiratory viral infections include respiratory syncytial virus (RSV), rhinovirus, influenza, para influenza, and adenovirus which is RSV and influenza infection leading to decreases in lung function [41]. Also, viral respiratory infections show pronounced and long-lasting effects on patients with CF, resulting in significant declines in forced vital capacity (FVC), forced expiratory volume in 1 second (FEV-1), and significant increases of both the frequency and duration of hospitalizations especially that the frequency of viral respiratory infections is closely associated with pulmonary deterioration in patients with CF [42]. Additionally, viral respiratory infections occur in equal frequency in CF patients and healthy controls which in CF patients viral upper respiratory tract infections are associated with lower respiratory tract symptoms in 31–76%. Viral infections cause long-term respiratory morbidity in CF patients [43].

7. Prevention and control of microorganisms in cystic fibrosis

Despite the development of antibiotics and vaccines, patients with CF are still faced with many debilitating and fatal infections, which demonstrate the adaptability of microbial pathogens [44]. The choice of antibiotic depends on in vitro sensitivity patterns. Physicians treating patients with CF are increasingly faced with infection with multidrug-resistant strains of *Pseudomonas aeruginosa*. Also, innately resistant organisms such as *Burkholderia cepacia*, *Stenotrophomonas maltophilia*, and *Achromobacter xylosoxidans* become more prevalent [45].

Additionally, many studies resulted in strong indicator for a relevant importance of mutators in bacterial populations especially in infectious diseases. High prevalence and mutators are recorded environmentally in chronic respiratory infection with *Pseudomonas aeruginosa* in CF patients [46].

7.1 Strategies and guidelines for bacterial infection control within CF patients

Guidelines on infection control developed for general patient populations are applicable to CF patients. Historically, before 1998, guidelines on infection control were applied to acute-care hospitals. Recently it includes for non-acute-care settings. Also, it has shifted from hospitals to home and outpatient clinics to reduce days of hospitalization and provide chronic suppressive treatments. Infection control in CF guidelines has been developed by Healthcare Infection Control Practices Advisory Committee (HICPAC) and Centers for Disease Control and Prevention (CDC) [47].

Common pathogens that infect the lungs of CF patients include *Staphylococcus aureus*, *Haemophilus influenzae*, *Pseudomonas aeruginosa*, and *Burkholderia cepacia*. Aggressively treating pulmonary infection with antibiotics has contributed to improved survival in patients with CF but has also promoted multiple drug-resistant bacteria [48].

Antibiotic therapy leads to improvement in lung function, the best predictor of survival in CF patients which treat CF lung disease morbidity based on decisions with which antibiotics are selected according to broad empirical and based on the severity of the patient's pulmonary exacerbation, the colonizing microorganisms, and the patient's age [49].

A range of anaerobic bacterial species are present in huge numbers in the lungs of CF patients, which contribute significantly to infection and inflammation in the CF lung. So, informed alterations of antibiotic treatment to target anaerobes is done, in addition to the primary infecting pathogens, may improve management [50].

A positive approach to the protection of the lung from early in life seems to be the only way to change the slope of the survival curves [51]. Ticarcillin can be used in the treatment of pulmonary exacerbations of cystic fibrosis due to susceptible strains of *Pseudomonas aeruginosa* [52, 53].

Also, *Alcaligenes* bacterial strains are characterized as motile, Gram-negative, producing oxidase enzyme. The most common is *Alcaligenes xylosoxidans* known as *Achromobacter xylosoxidans*. The bacterial genus is composed of three main species such as *Achromobacter piechaudii*, *Achromobacter xylosoxidans*, and *Achromobacter faecalis.* These bacterial strains observed multiple antibiotic resistance especially grouped of aminoglycosides and recorded sensitivity to cephalosporins (third generation) [54].

7.2 Inhalational antibiotics for the treatment of *Pseudomonas aeruginosa*

In recent years, there are emergences of inhaled antibiotics to treat patients with Gram-negative bacterial infection such as *P. aeruginosa* infection. The benefits of which are explained below [55, 56].

Inhaled tobramycin, inhaled colistin, and inhaled aztreonam are used to control chronic *P. aeruginosa* infections in patients with CF [57]. In CF, tobramycin inhalation solution contributed to improved survival and reduced lung function decline [58]. Subsequently, the development of antibiotic agents can achieve high tissue concentrations to control bacterial infection that is difficult to treat in hosts [59]. Inhaled tobramycin achieves a sputum concentration of drug at least 25 times the MIC, with a median serum/sputum concentration of 0.01. Such high concentrations are required for the effective killing of *P. aeruginosa* because aminoglycosides bind to mucins in sputum and reduce the availability of effective antibiotic. Also, early randomized, double-blind, placebo-controlled trials conducted in patients with CF were short-term but demonstrated positive results with the use of aztreonam solution for inhalation compared to placebo. Colistin is bactericidal and active against Gram-negative bacteria including *P. aeruginosa*. Nebulized colistin is a preferred inhaled therapy for patients with CF and chronic *P. aeruginosa* [59]. Inhaled levofloxacin was studied in patients with CF and *P. aeruginosa* lung infection. Also, nebulized levofloxacin solution (MP-376) is a novel therapy that is currently being evaluated in phase I, II, and III clinical trials among patients with stable CF and recent isolation of *Pseudomonas aeruginosa* from sputum [60].

7.3 Antifungal therapy to control yeasts and filamentous fungi with CF patients

Antifungal therapy is usually considered when the deteriorating respiratory function is not responding to antibacterial therapy and *A. fumigatus* is growing and identified in sputum cultures [61]. Long-term antifungal treatment with mold active azoles, the only class of antifungals with an oral formulation, is not without risk of toxicity and adverse events and should be carefully balanced against its benefit [10].

A. fumigatus can grow in sputum cultures, and antifungal therapy is not effective [61]. Also, *Scedosporium* sp. is the second most frequent cystic fibrosis associated filamentous fungi which is resistant to many antifungal agents [62].

In CF, *Candida albicans* causes 95% of all *Candida* infections, whereas the remainder is caused by *Candida glabrata*, *Candida parapsilosis*, and *Candida krusei*. Also, *Candida dubliniensis* has been isolated in CF; however, little is known about its potential for virulence, and treatment modality is not clearly defined [63].

7.4 Antiviral therapy to control respiratory viruses with CF patients

Respiratory viruses associated with exacerbations in CF patients and upper respiratory symptoms are strong predictors for their presence. Some studies have suggested a role played by respiratory viruses in exacerbation of CF. The impact of respiratory viruses is likely to be underestimated due to the low detection rate by conventional laboratory methods. Molecular techniques such as multiplex PCR have improved their diagnostic accuracy identifying respiratory viruses in CF patients which are important in clinical decision-making and are potentially important as new antivirals are becoming readily available [64]. A few therapeutic options recorded to treat virus-induced CF pulmonary exacerbations include macrolide antibiotic (azithromycin). It has antiviral properties of the human bronchial epithelial cells and stimulates antiviral mechanisms in bronchial epithelial cells within the CF airway control infection with rhinovirus by reducing rhinovirus replication as an interferon pathway [65]. Also, there are exciting prospects such as antiviral host defense peptides in development and can be novel therapeutics targeting rhinovirus [66].

Additionally, CF patients infected with influenza A(H1N1) showed increased case fatality rate (CFR) and morbidity compared to patients with other chronic respiratory diseases, so, early antibiotic and antiviral treatment strategies are important to control it in CF patients [67].

8. Conclusion

This chapter concludes that complications of microorganisms associated with cystic fibrosis disease are very high and can lead to patient death. Pathogenic microorganisms isolated from CF patients included Gram-negative bacteria, Gram-positive bacteria, unicellular fungi, multicellular fungi, and viruses.

The most common Gram-negative bacterial pathogens are *Pseudomonas aeruginosa* and *Haemophilus influenzae*. Also, the most common Gram-positive bacterial pathogen is *Staphylococcus aureus* especially MRSA. Other bacterial pathogens are isolated from CF patients, such as NTM species, *Alcaligenes xylosoxidans*, and *Burkholderia cenocepacia*.

In addition, *Candida albicans* is the most common unicellular fungi, and *Aspergillus fumigatus* is the most common filamentous fungi. Influenza A and B viruses are major viruses in causing respiratory exacerbations in CF, and both viruses are more commonly detected during pulmonary exacerbations.

To prevent this microbial complication, appropriate antimicrobials can be used to treat bacterial infections, antifungal therapy for treating pathogenic fungi and antiviral to manage viral infections. With prospects, researchers must work to produce new therapeutic options to control multidrug-resistant bacteria and resistant fungi and virus. These new treatment options may further enhance the prognosis in patients with CF.

Acknowledgements

Firstly, great thanks and appreciation to Prof. Dr. Mamdouh Salem Elgamal and Prof. Dr. Ayman Farrag Ahmed for their support and encouragement. Finally, I wish to thank my mother, brother, sisters, children (Khalid and Mohammed), and everyone in my family for their continual guidance.

Conflict of interest

The author declares no conflict of interest.

Abbreviations

CF	cystic fibrosis
CFTR	cystic fibrosis transmembrane conductance regulator gene
MRSA	methicillin-resistant *Staphylococcus aureus*
NTM	nontuberculous mycobacteria
CFR	case fatality rate

Author details

Salah Abdelbary
Botany and Microbiology Department, Faculty of Science, Al-Azhar University, Cairo, Egypt

*Address all correspondence to: salah.micro87@gmail.com; abdelbary_salah@azhar.edu.eg

References

[1] Biology C, Chotirmall SH, Mcelvaney NG. Fungi in the cystic fibrosis lung: Bystanders or pathogens. The International Journal of Biochemistry & Cell Biology. 2014;**52**:161-173

[2] Lobo J, Rojas-balcazar JM, Noone PG. Recent advances in cystic fibrosis. Clinics in Chest Medicine. 1989;**33**(2):307-328

[3] Bowen S, Hull J. The basic science of cystic fibrosis. Paediatrics & Child Health. 2015;**25**(4):159-164

[4] Fre E. The airway microbiota in cystic fibrosis: A complex fungal and bacterial community. Implications for Therapeutic Management. 2012;**7**(4): 1-14. https://doi.org/10.1371/journal.pone.0036313

[5] Santana MA, Matos E. Prevalence of pathogens in cystic fibrosis patients in Bahia, Brazil. Brazilian Journal of Infectious Diseases. 2003;**7**:69-72

[6] Cribbs SK, Beck JM. Microbiome in the pathogenesis of cystic fibrosis and lung transplant-related disease. Translational Research. 2016;**179**:84-96

[7] Tang AC, Turvey SE, Alves MP, Regamey N, Tu B, Hartl D. Current concepts: Host – Pathogen interactions in cystic fibrosis airways disease. European Respiratory Review. 2014;(133):320-332. DOI: 10.1183/09059180.00006113

[8] Godoy JM, Godoy AN, Ribalta G, Largo I. Bacterial Pattern in Chronic Sinusitis and Cystic Fibrosis. Otolaryngology-Head and Neck Surgery. Oct 2011;**145**(4):673-676. DOI: 10.1177/0194599811407279

[9] Hector A et al. Microbial colonization and lung function in adolescents with cystic fibrosis. Journal of Cystic Fibrosis. 2016;**15**:340-349. DOI: 10.1016/j.jcf.2016.01.004

[10] King J, Brunel SF, Warris A. Aspergillus infections in cystic fibrosis. The Journal of Infection. 2016;**72**:S50-S55

[11] Rowe SM, Hoover MW, Solomon GM, Sorscher EJ. 47 - Cystic Fibrosis. Sixth Edn: Elsevier Inc.; 1948

[12] Folkesson A et al. Adaptation of Pseudomonas aeruginosa to the cystic fibrosis airway: An evolutionary perspective. Nature Publishing Group. 2012;**10**(12):841-851

[13] Waters V, Smyth A. Cystic fibrosis microbiology: Advances in antimicrobial therapy. Journal of Cystic Fibrosis. 2015;**14**(5):551-560

[14] Molina SA, Hunt WR. Cystic Fibrosis: An Overview of the Past, Present, and the Future. Lung Epithelial Biology in the Pathogenesis of Pulmonary Disease. 2017:219-249. https://doi.org/10.1016/B978-0-12-803809-3.00012-9

[15] Lobo LJ, Noone PG. Respiratory infections in patients with cystic fibrosis undergoing lung transplantation. The Lancet Respiratory Medicine. 2014;**2**(1):73-82

[16] Hauser PM, Bernard T, Greub G, Jaton K, Pagni M, Hafen GM. Microbiota present in cystic fibrosis lungs as revealed by whole genome sequencing. PLoS One. 5 Mar 2014;**9**(3):e90934. DOI: 10.1371/journal.pone.0090934

[17] Döring G. Prevention of *Pseudomonas aeruginosa* infection in cystic fibrosis patients. International Journal of Medical Microbiology. 2010;**300**:573-577

[18] Sousa AM, Monteiro R, Pereira MO. International journal of

medical microbiology unveiling the early events of Pseudomonas aeruginosa adaptation in cystic fibrosis airway environment using a long-term in vitro maintenance. International Journal of Medical Microbiology. 2018;**308**(8):1053-1064

[19] Field TR, Sibley CD, Parkins MD, Rabin HR, Surette MG. Anaerobe the genus Prevotella in cystic fibrosis airways. Anaerobe. 2010;**16**(4):337-344

[20] Rodríguez-sevilla G et al. International journal of medical microbiology non-Tuberculous mycobacteria multispecies bio films in cystic fibrosis: Development of an in vitro Mycobacterium abscessus and Pseudomonas aeruginosa dual species bio fi lm model. International Journal of Medical Microbiology. 2018;**308**(3):413-423

[21] Martin C et al. Host–microbe interactions in distal airways: Relevance to chronic airway diseases. European Respiratory Review. 2015;**24**(135):78-91

[22] Hector A, Frey N, Hartl D. Update on host-pathogen interactions in cystic fibrosis lung disease. Molecular and Cellular Pediatrics. 2016;**3**(1):12

[23] Yonker LM, Cigana C, Hurley BP, Bragonzi A. Host-pathogen interplay in the respiratory environment of cystic fibrosis. Journal of Cystic Fibrosis. 2015;**14**(4):431-439

[24] Floto RA, Olivier KN, Saiman L, Daley CL, Herrmann J, Nick JA, et al. US Cystic Fibrosis Foundation and European cystic fibrosis society consensus recommendations for the management of non-tuberculous mycobacteria in individuals with cystic fibrosis. Thorax. 2016;**71**:i1-i22

[25] Furukawa BS, Flume PA. Nontuberculous mycobacteria in cystic fibrosis. Seminars in Respiratory and Critical Care Medicine. 2018 Jun;**39**(3):383-391

[26] Mussaffi H, Rivlin J, Shalit I, Ephros M, Blau H. Nontuberculous mycobacteria in cystic fibrosis associated with allergic bronchopulmonary aspergillosis and steroid therapy. European Respiratory Journal. 2005;**25**:324-328

[27] Govan JR, Deretic V. Microbial pathogenesis in cystic fibrosis: Mucoid Pseudomonas aeruginosa and Burkholderia cepacia. Microbiological Reviews. 1996;**60**:539-574

[28] Li Z, Kosorok MR, Farrell PM. Longitudinal development of mucoid Pseudomonas aeruginosa infection and lung disease progression in children with cystic fibrosis. JAMA. 2005;**293**:581-588

[29] Berry A, JD DV, Chakrabarty AM. High osmolarity is a signal for enhanced algD transcription in mucoid and nonmucoid Pseudomonas aeruginosa strains. Journal of Bacteriology. 1989;**171**:2312-2317

[30] Fegan M, Francis P, Hayward AC. Phenotypic conversion of Pseudomonas aeruginosa in cystic fibrosis. Journal of Clinical Microbiology. 1990;**28**:1143-1146

[31] Govan JR, Harris GS. Pseudomonas aeruginosa and cystic fibrosis: Unusual bacterial adaptation and pathogenesis. Microbiological Sciences. 1986;**3**:302-308

[32] Lam J, Chan R, Lam K, et al. Production of mucoid microcolonies by Pseudomonas aeruginosa within infected lungs in cystic fibrosis. Infection and Immunity. 1980;**28**:546-556

[33] Pier GB, Coleman F, Grout M. Role of alginate O acetylation in resistance of mucoid Pseudomonas

aeruginosa to opsonic phagocytosis. Infection and Immunity. 2001;**69**:1895-1901

[34] Ciofu O, Fussing V, Bagge N. Characterization of paired mucoid/non-mucoid Pseudomonas aeruginosa isolates from Danish cystic fibrosis patients: Antibiotic resistance, betalactamase activity and RiboPrinting. The Journal of Antimicrobial Chemotherapy. 2001;**48**:391-396

[35] Alma L. "Bacterial colonization in cystic fibrosis" very well health. Cystic Fibrosis. 2018;(2):1-7

[36] Pittman JE, Calloway EH. Age of Pseudomonas aeruginosa acquisition and subsequent severity of cystic fibrosis lung disease. Pediatric Pulmonology. 2011;**46**(5):497-504

[37] Hauser AR, Jain M, Bar-meir M, Mccolley SA. Clinical significance of microbial infection and adaptation in cystic fibrosis. Clinical Microbiology Reviews. 2011;**24**(1):29-70. DOI: 10.1128/CMR.00036-10

[38] Gilligan PH. Infections in patients with cystic fibrosis diagnostic microbiology update infection cystic fibrosis diagnostic microbiology update. Clinics in Laboratory Medicine. Jun 2014;**34**(2):197-217. DOI: 10.1016/j.cll.2014.02.001

[39] Saiman L. Infection Prevention and Control in Cystic Fibrosis. Current Opinion in Infectious Diseases. Aug 2011;**24**(4):390-395. DOI: 10.1097/QCO.0b013e32834748ff

[40] Janahi IA. Abdul Rehman and Amal Rashid Al-Naimi, allergic bronchopulmonary aspergillosis in patients with cystic fibrosis. Annals of Thoracic Medicine. 2017;**12**(2):74-82

[41] Megan R, Jennifer M. Viral-bacterial co-infections in the cystic fibrosis respiratory tract. Frontiers in Immunology. 2018;**9**:3067. DOI: 10.3389/fimmu.2018.03067

[42] Frickmann H, Jungblut S, Hirche TO, Groß U, Kuhns M, Zautner AE. Spectrum of viral infections in patients with cystic fibrosis. European Journal of Microbiology and Immunology. 2012;**2**(3):161-175. DOI: 10.1556/EuJMI.2.2012.3.1

[43] Bart E, Marieke M, Tom FW, Cornelis van der Enta K. Viral respiratory infections in cystic fibrosis. Journal of Cystic Fibrosis. 2005;**4**:31-36

[44] Hoiby N. Microbiology of lung infection in CF patients. Acta Paediatrica Scandinavica. Supplement. 1982;**301**(4):33-54

[45] Conway SP, Brownlee KG, Denton M, Peckham DG. Antibiotic treatment of multidrug-resistant organisms in cystic fibrosis organisms in cystic fibrosis. American Journal of Respiratory Medicine. 2003;**2**(4):321-332

[46] Oliver A, Mena A. Bacterial hypermutation in cystic fibrosis, not only for antibiotic resistance. Clinical Microbiology and Infection. 2010;**16**(7):798-808

[47] Govan JRW. Infection control in cystic fibrosis: Methicillin-resistant Staphylococcus aureus, Pseudomonas aeruginosa and the Burkholderia cepacia complex. Journal of the Royal Society of Medicine. 2000;**93**(38):40-45

[48] O'Malley CA. Infection control in cystic fibrosis: Cohorting, cross-contamination, and the respiratory therapist introduction Care of Respiratory Equipment. Respiratory Care. 2009;**54**(5):641-657

[49] Lyczak JB, Cannon CL, Pier GB. Lung infections associated with cystic fibrosis. Clinical Microbiology Reviews. 2002;**15**(2):194-222

[50] Tunney MM et al. Detection of anaerobic bacteria in high numbers in sputum from patients with cystic fibrosis. American Journal of Respiratory and Critical Care Medicine. 2008;**177**(9):995-1001

[51] Elborn JS, Shale DJ. Cystic fibrosis: 2 - lung injury in cystic fibrosis. Thorax. 1990;**45**(12):970-973

[52] Parry MF, Neu HC, Merlino M, Gaerlan PF, Ores CN, Denning CR. Treatment of pulmonary infections in patients with cystic fibrosis: A comparative study of ticarcillin and gentamicin. The Journal of Pediatrics. 1977;**90**(1):144-148

[53] Harrison F. Microbial ecology of the cystic fibrosis lung. Microbiology. 2007;**153**(4):917-923

[54] Tan K, Conway SP, Brownlee KG, Etherington C, Peckham DG. Alcaligenes infection in cystic fibrosis. Pediatric Pulmonology. 2002;**34**(2):101-104

[55] Wenzler E, Fraidenburg DR, Scardina T, Danziger LH. Inhaled antibiotics for gram-negative respiratory infections. Clinical Microbiology Reviews. 2016;**29**(3):581-632

[56] Sabet M, Miller CE, Nolan TG, Senekeo-Effenberger K, Dudley MN, Griffith DC. Efficacy of aerosol MP-376, a levofloxacin inhalation solution, in models of mouse lung infection due to Pseudomonas aeruginosa. Antimicrobial Agents and Chemotherapy. 2009;**53**(9):3923-3928

[57] Anderson G, Akhand S, Pettit R, Gardner T. New treatments in development for Pseudomonas aeruginosa infections in the lungs of individuals with cystic fibrosis. Orphan Drugs: Research and Reviews. 2014;**4**:71

[58] P. M.D. and E. J.S. Tobramycin inhalation PowderTM: A novel drug delivery system for treating chronic Pseudomonas aeruginosa infection in cystic fibrosis. Expert Review of Respiratory Medicine. 2011;**5**(5):609-622

[59] Maselli DJ, Keyt H, Restrepo MI. Inhaled antibiotic therapy in chronic respiratory diseases. International Journal of Molecular Sciences. 2017;**18**(5):1-23. DOI: 10.3390/ijms18051062

[60] Stockmann C, Sherwin CM, Ampofo K, Spigarelli MG. Development of levofloxacin inhalation solution to treat *Pseudomonas aeruginosa* in patients with cystic fibrosis. Therapeutic Advances in Respiratory Disease. 2014;**8**(1):13-21. DOI: 10.1177/1753465813508445

[61] Shoseyov D, Brownlee KG, Conway SP, Kerem E. Aspergillus bronchitis in cystic fibrosis. Chest. 2006;**130**(1):222-226

[62] Blyth CC, Middleton PG, Harun A, Sorrell TC, Meyer W, Chen SCA. Clinical associations and prevalence of Scedosporium spp. in Australian cystic fibrosis patients: Identification of novel risk factors? Medical Mycology. 2010;**48**(O1):37-44

[63] Chotirmall SH, O'Donoghue E, Bennett K, Gunaratnam C, O'Neill SJ, McElvaney NG. Sputum Candida albicans presages FEV1decline and hospital-treated exacerbations in cystic fibrosis. Chest. 2010;**138**(5):1186-1195

[64] Wat D et al. The role of respiratory viruses in cystic fibrosis. Journal of Cystic Fibrosis. 2008;**7**(4):320-328

[65] Schögler A et al. Novel antiviral properties of azithromycin in cystic fibrosis airway epithelial cells. The European Respiratory Journal. 2015;**45**(2):428-439

[66] Casanova V, Sousa FH, Stevens C, Barlow PG. Antiviral therapeutic approaches for human rhinovirus infections. Future Virology. 2018;**13**(7):505-518

[67] Renk H, Regamey N, Hartl D. Influenza a(H1N1)pdm09 and cystic fibrosis lung disease: A systematic meta-analysis. PLoS One. 2014;**9**(1):e93142, 1-2. DOI: 10.1371/journal.pone.0093142

Chapter 3

Overview of CFTR Modulators and Gene Therapy

Catherine Rang, Tom Kotsimbos and John Wilson

Abstract

Individuals with cystic fibrosis (CF) have seen a substantial change in their life expectancy since the introduction of coordinated multi-disciplinary care. This is expected to continue with the recent availability of treatment options that focus on targeting the underlying genetic defect. Two different approaches to altering the consequence of mutations in the cystic fibrosis transmembrane conductance regulator (CFTR) gene include "genetic medicines", in particular gene therapy, and CFTR modulator agents. Gene therapy requires further development prior to it being a treatment option because to date the best clinical outcomes are that of a reduction in the rate of lung function decline. Modulator therapies on the other hand have provided exciting results in both clinical trials and real-world settings. Potentiator agents alter dysfunctional ion channel gating and are suitable for gating mutations. Corrector agents target abnormal protein trafficking. The combination of potentiator and corrector therapy provides options for homozygotes with the commonest mutation Phe508del and for those with Phe508del and some residual function mutations. Newer modulator therapies are in continued development with progressively impressive outcomes. It is likely that future CF care will comprise of personalized strategies with the focus centered upon an individual's specific mutations.

Keywords: cystic fibrosis, CF pathophysiology, CFTR modulator therapy, gene therapy

1. Introduction

Cystic fibrosis (CF) is an autosomal recessive condition that results from mutations in the cystic fibrosis transmembrane conductor regulator (CFTR) gene located on the long arm of chromosome 7. The gene was identified 30 years ago and since then over 2000 CFTR mutations have been discovered with more than 300 known to be disease causing [1, 2]. The commonest mutation is Phe508del (F508del; c.1521_1523delCTT), where a phenylalanine is substituted at position 508 on chromosome 7. Worldwide approximately 80–90% of individuals with CF have at least one copy of the Phe508del-CFTR mutation, although mutation rates varying depending upon the population cohort [3–5].

CF is a multi-system disease with the highest disease prevalence being in Europe, North America and Australia. There are approximately 80,000 people with CF worldwide. The disease is characterized by chronic airway infection, pancreatic insufficiency and malnutrition, diabetes, liver disease, absent vas deferens and premature death.

Due to the multi-system nature of the disease, treatment has classically focused on therapies and systems of care that aim to improve salt and fluid balance and nutritional status, alongside reducing airway inflammation and lung parenchymal destruction. These multi-disciplinary management approaches have been instrumental in the improvements seen in life expectancy. The median predicated survival of an individual born today with CF is 47 years, compared with 20 years at the time when CFTR was discovered in 1989 [2]. However, to have a true impact upon the management of these patients and to alter the disease trajectory, treatment options needed to also include approaches targeting the underlying genetic mutation.

This chapter will include a review of the structure of the CFTR protein, its biosynthesis and the pathophysiology of CF so as to provide a basis from which to discuss the various therapeutic strategies that have more recently been developed for modulating CFTR protein function. Also, a discussion regarding gene therapy will be included so as to enable contrasts and comparisons to be made between the different therapies being evolved to address the underlying genetic defect in CF patients.

2. Pathophysiology of cystic fibrosis

2.1 CFTR protein structure

CFTR codes for a complex protein, which is present in every nucleated cell of the body, however it is normally concentrated on the apical membrane of epithelial cells, primarily within the glandular epithelia. High expression of this apical anion channel is seen within the lungs, pancreas, gastrointestinal tract, vas deferens and sweat glands; reflecting the main organs affected in CF [6].

The CFTR protein is a large, unique member of the subclass C family of the ATP binding cassette (ABC) transporter proteins, which functions as an ion channel rather than an active transporter protein [7–9]. It consists of two membrane-spanning domains (MBDs) that form the ion channel. These domains are both connected to two cytoplasmic nucleotide-binding domains (NBD1 and NBD2), which function to gate the channel. This conformation of two MBDs and two NBDs that hydrolyse ATP are typical for most ABC transporters. However, CFTR has an additional cytoplasmic regulatory domain (R domain), inserted between NBD1 and MSD2 linking the two transporter domains. Phosphorylation of the R domain by protein kinase A enables channel opening to occur and channel activity is increased upon phosphorylation. Once phosphorylation has taken place, ATP binds to the NBDs resulting in the two NBDs forming tightly interacting dimers, which gates the channel. These movements are transmitted to the MBDs causing the ion pore to open. Channel closure results from ATP hydrolysis. The exact mechanisms underlying the regulation of the R domain and ATP-dependent gating are still not completely understood [10, 11].

2.2 CFTR protein synthesis

CFTR protein synthesis is a complex process, in part related to the size of the functional protein. As with all protein synthesis, transcription of the CFTR DNA takes place within the nucleus to create the messenger RNA (mRNA), which is transported across the nuclear membrane to the cytosolic ribosomes. There the initiation of translation occurs to create a 1480-amino acid polypeptide chain based upon the genetic code. Initially a 135- to 140-kDa core-glycosylated precursor is produced (immature CFTR). CFTR biosynthesis then proceeds through the endoplasmic reticulum (ER) followed by the Golgi apparatus to a mature 150- to 160-kDa CFTR form which has undergone conformational folding [12]. During the secretory pathway through the ER to the Golgi and then on to the cell membrane various post-translational modifications take place (**Figure 1**).

The maturation process to create the final relatively compact CFTR protein structure is inefficient and slow. Less than 30% of newly synthesized wild-type (wt) immature CFTR molecules develop into mature CFTR proteins. For folding of the polypeptide chain to occur chaperones are required, in particular the 70 k-Da heat shock proteins (HSP70) and calnexin. In cells of individuals with the Phe508del-CFTR mutation, almost all immature molecules fail to reach final maturity and thus are degraded. This is the due to the quality control mechanisms in place within the ER, specific signals and distinct processes exist that recruit misfolded proteins to the ER-associated degradation as a final endpoint. These proteins are then directed for degradation via the ubiquitin-proteasome pathway [12–14] (**Figure 1**).

Certain steps within the CFTR biosynthesis pathway are still unknown, however, data does support each domain folding independently. The native structure develops through a co-translational mechanism, possibly together with post-translational processes that take place to create the compactly folded domains. Domain-domain interactions are key in the creation of conformationally correct CFTR [15]. Furthermore, it appears that CFTR is more sensitive to mutations in NBD1 compared with homologous mutations in NBD2, leading to issues with the conformational maturation of the whole CFTR protein. For example, the deletion of the Phe508 does not appear to grossly alter the structure of NBD1 but subsequent issues arise during the maturation process, possibly through the disruption of the interaction between NBD1 and NBD2 and despite each domain folding independently. Maturation thus requires precise folding of each domain together with the

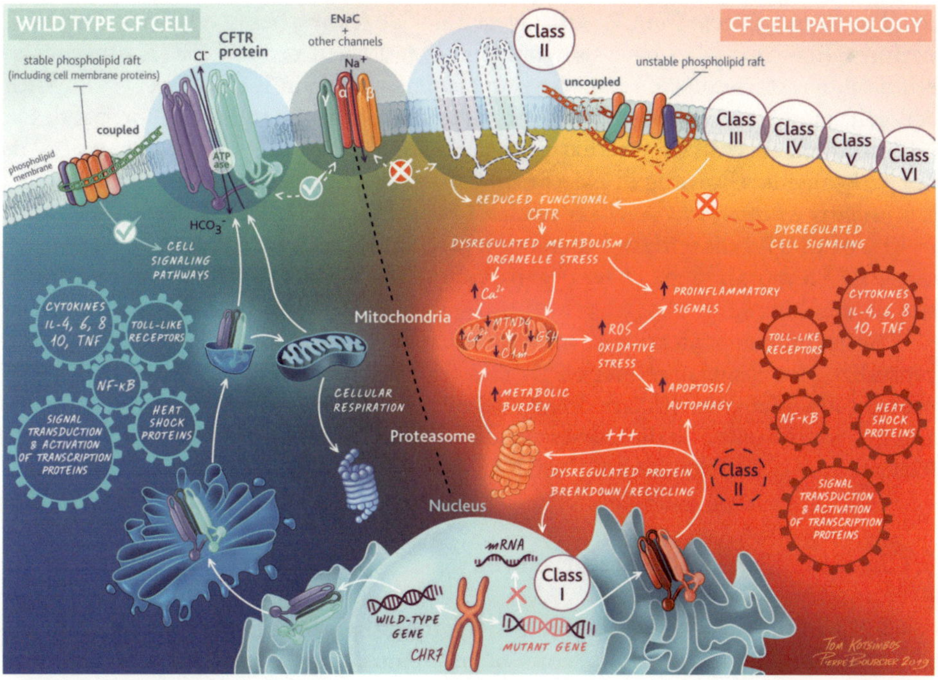

Figure 1.
Cell biology of CFTR - abnormal CFTR protein results in the uncoupling of CFTR dependent processes at all levels from intracellular dynamics to cell membrane function. Reproduced with permission of the © ERS 2020: European Respiratory Journal; DOI: 10.1183/13993003.02443-2019: Accepted for publication and in press.

correct inter-domain assembly to create a stable structure that will not be submitted to ER-associated degradation [13, 16].

If the protein passes through all the checkpoint steps within the ER, it can exit and be transported through the Golgi apparatus in vesicles where the removal and addition of new glycan units takes place, increasing the molecular size of CFTR. It is becoming clear that some wt-CFTR might bypass these processes in the delivery pathway to the plasma membrane. Once at the membrane, levels of CFTR vary depending upon the balance of anterograde trafficking, endocytosis and recycling. Recycling of internalized CFTR to the plasma membrane is thought to assist with sustaining a functional pool of CFTR at the membrane level [15].

2.3 Pathophysiology

CFTR functions as a chloride and bicarbonate channel. Loss of functional CFTR proteins result in reduced chloride efflux from epithelial cells leading to depletion of the cell surface fluid and altering its pH and osmolarity. CFTR also regulates the activity of various other key processes within the cell, including the activity of other ion channels, such as the sodium epithelial channel (ENaC; the amiloride-sensitive sodium channel). Suppressed CFTR activity can lead to unopposed reabsorption of sodium and water via ENaC, causing additional dehydration of the cell surface layer [6]. Mucociliary clearance is further delayed due to abnormally adherent mucus. Dysfunctional CFTR also impacts upon mitochondrial function, the innate immunity and dysregulates inflammation [17–19]. Within the airways, this results in an environment that is susceptible to unchecked inflammation and chronic bacterial infection.

Although multiple processes both intra- and extra-cellularly are altered by dysfunctional CFTR proteins, chloride transport at the cell surface is generally considered to be the major driver of the pathophysiological disease. Functional chloride channel changes are thus likely to represent an easily accessible surrogate marker of all processes affected in CF, with sweat chloride testing being relatively easy to perform. In vitro studies have shown that only 6–10% of residual CFTR function is required to restore chloride transporting properties seen in 100% correct cells, with cell-cell coupling providing a means of amplification of the functional properties [20]. Individuals with CF who have approximately 10% CTFR expression per cell do not generally develop lung disease or the full range of classical CF disease. To date, it is unclear whether low level expression (10%) of CFTR in all cells is comparable to 10% of CFTR cells with full correction [21]. In addition, even individuals with a single CFTR mutation may have organ dysfunction in the context of a second "hit" such as smoking [22].

The general identification of mutations in the structure of CFTR has been centralized for clinician reference. CFTR2.org identifies over 2000 variants of the protein, of which over 400 are disease-associated. The majority of variants are rare and not confirmed to be disease-associated, however the large number of variants indicates the lack of stability of the CFTR gene in population dynamics [1].

3. Classification of CFTR mutations

Classification systems of common CFTR mutations have been developed to assist with understanding of the consequential molecular defect. The established classification system includes six different classes (**Figure 2**). Different mutations can result in no functional protein production, impaired protein trafficking, altered channel gating, decreased channel conductance, reduced protein synthesis and decreased protein stability [6]. Each class confers a different disease severity, which

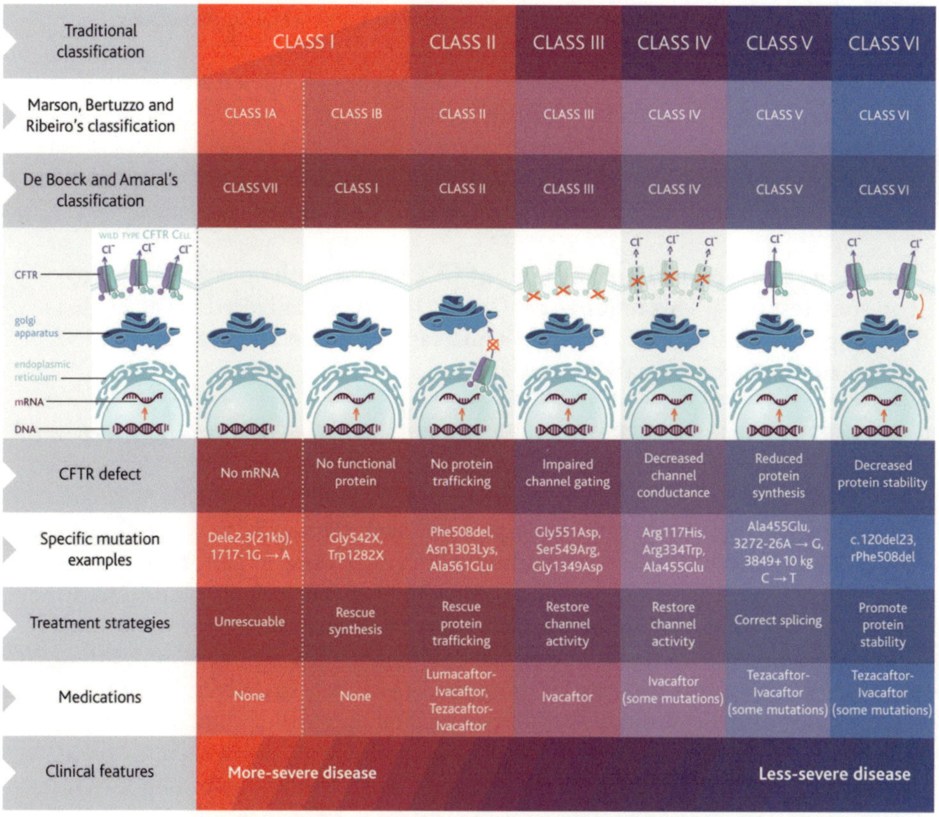

Figure 2.
CFTR classification table. The classification systems divide mutations into discrete groups determined by the predominant CFTR defect. However, these systems may not be mutually exclusive for all mutations. For example, the p.Phe508del-CFTR is predominately class II but does also have some class III and class VI properties. Reproduced with permission of the © ERS 2020: European Respiratory Journal; DOI: 10.1183/13993003.02443-2019: Accepted for publication and in press.

is related to the degree of CFTR dysfunction and has prognostic implications for patients. However, each mutation may have features of more than just one class. For example, Phe508del is predominately a class II mutation but also has both class III and class VI properties. More recently, other classification systems have been proposed, which subdivide class I mutations (no functional CFTR protein) into two groups so as to take into account whether the mutation leads to no mRNA or no functional protein [23].

4. Genetic medicines

Traditional CF care has focused upon the management of the systems affected in individuals with CF. However, the identification of the CFTR gene enabled researchers to focus on treatments strategies, which could address the underlying genetic defect. The major cause of morbidity and mortality in CF is secondary to lung disease. Hence, if abnormal CFTR in the lungs could be replaced with wt-CFTR during the neonatal period, prior to parenchymal lung damage or bacterial colonization, morbidity and mortality could be significantly altered within the CF population [24]. Various approaches have been investigated within the field of "genetic medicines" and unfortunately to date none are a viable treatment option outside of clinical trials.

"Genetic medicines" comprise of four different treatment approaches:

i. **Gene therapy:** the delivery of wt-CFTR to the cell nucleus resulting in the production of normal CFTR protein;

ii. **mRNA therapy:** the delivery of correct CFTR mRNA to the cytoplasm resulting in the production of normal CFTR protein;

iii. **Gene editing:** repair of the mutant CFTR DNA with normal CFTR protein resulting. This requires wt-CFTR DNA to be delivered to the nucleus together with mRNA encoding a nuclease that causes a break in the DNA leading to recombination occurring;

iv. **mRNA editing:** CFTR mRNA delivery to the cytoplasm leading to repair of the CFTR mRNA [21].

The potential benefit of these therapies is that theoretically they should be suitable for the treatment of all individuals with CF, regardless of genotype. Currently gene therapy has made the greatest advancement towards being a clinical treatment and so the main focus of this section will be around gene therapy.

As the respiratory system is so central to CF disease and because initial thoughts were that gene therapy targeting the lungs would be easy to deliver, locally directed gene therapy to the respiratory epithelium was the method of choice. Furthermore, gene therapy can complement any CFTR causing mutation. However, for such treatment to be successful various issues had to be addressed, including the choice of delivery vector, method of delivery to the airways, translocation of the genetic information and ultimately ensuring that there was appropriate expression of the normalized CFTR gene [25]. These various issues will each be discussed to provide insight in the difficulties experienced in trying to develop "genetic medicines."

The lungs are comprised of terminally differentiated epithelial cells, which are slowly replaced by stem/progenitor cells. Any form of gene therapy must be able to be either repeatedly delivered to the terminally-differentiated cell surface or be able to alter the stem/progenitor cells within the lungs. However, the lung has evolved physical and immune mechanisms to protect against pathogens and particulate materials, which impacts upon choice of vector delivery [26, 27].

Delivery vectors are largely either viral or non-viral in nature with viral ones felt to be more efficient. This is because they have evolved to overcome the barrier mechanisms present within the lungs. Adenoviruses (Ad) and adeno-associated viruses (AAV) have a natural trophism for the lungs, are DNA-based and thus were the initial choices to study. Adenoviruses are small in size and thus to insert the CFTR DNA correctly within the adenoviral genome, viral DNA must be removed, impacting upon the viral cytopathic effect. These vectors were found to have poor efficacy due to the pre-existing and induced immune responses, and thus cannot be repeatedly administered as required for these treatments because of the short life span of bronchial epithelial cells.

Other viral vectors that have been investigated are recombinant lentivirus (rLV). These agents are RNA-based and can integrate into the genome. This can be advantageous as it ensures that the vector is passed down the cell lines during division but it also does have the risk of inducing insertional mutagenesis [21, 26, 28]. However, ultimately other vectors were needed to be formulated, ones which had a minimal risk of immunogenicity and thus could be repeatedly administered.

Non-viral gene transfer agents complexed to plasmid DNA were therefore developed [21, 29]. These have been more successful than their viral vector counterparts and have been investigated in Phase IIb studies. Patients who were 12 years and older were treated with the non-viral CFTR gene-liposomal complex pGM169/GLG7A as a nebulized therapy over a one-year period. The repeated nebulization each month resulted in a reduction in the progression of CF lung disease by a modest amount when compared with placebo. The percentage change in the forced expiratory volume in 1 second (FEV_1) over 12 months was −0.4% versus −4.0% in the placebo arm. Hence, although no improvement in lung function was seen, this study was promising as rate of lung function decline does impact morbidity and mortality in CF. However, disappointingly also there were no improvements in quality of life measures [30].

As described in the above study the agents utilized were delivered via inhalation methods. This has been found to be the easiest method for repeated treatment applications. However, difficulties have arisen ensuring adequate lung deposition of drug, related to particle size and the type of nebulisers used. Additionally, any aerolised drug delivered must retain its biological function post-delivery [31, 32].

Other strategies for ensuring corrected CFTR protein production is through mRNA therapy and mRNA repair as described above. The benefit of these approaches is that they do not require translocation of the therapy across the nuclear membrane. Nanoparticle-chemically modified mRNA has resulted in lung function improvements in animal models without any immune reactions despite repeated applications. Also, there is evidence that these therapies can restore chloride channel activity [33, 34]. Ongoing work and investigation are required prior to these options being viable in the clinical setting.

5. CFTR modulator agents

CFTR modulator agents are small molecules which 'modulate' the function of the abnormal CFTR protein. Unlike gene therapy, they do not alter the CFTR gene. However, these agents do manipulate the underlying genetic consequence of CF mutations. Currently two different classes of modulator agents have been developed;

i. potentiators which 'potentiate' the cAMP-mediated gating of the CFTR channel; and

ii. correctors which 'correct' defects in protein trafficking.

5.1 CFTR modulator drug design

High-throughput drug discovery programs enabled the development of such agents. These discovery programs were established to identify active compounds ("hits") from large chemical libraries suitable for industrial-scale screening. High-throughput screening (HTS) assays need to be robust, have high throughput using small sample volumes together with adequate sensitivity, reproducibility and accuracy to ensure differentiation between a very large amount of compounds [35]. Ion channels are key targets for drug design and thus HTS have been an important part of such drug discovery processes, including for CF [36, 37].

The two classes of small molecules for CFTR protein modulation were identified via HTS techniques from libraries that consisted of chemically diverse drug-like and lead-like compounds acquired from both commercial vendors and internal medicine chemistry programs. If compounds had an activity >2.5 standard deviations (SD) from the mean, then they received further testing. For example, from

~164,000 synthetic compounds initial screened, approximately 100 were suitable for further study in one study [38]. The molecules identified were optimized and evaluated in terms of pharmacokinetics and toxicology [39, 40].

5.2 Potentiator therapy

The first small molecule clinically available for individuals with CF following HTS was Ivacaftor (Kalydeco®). It is an oral CFTR potentiator agent, which can be given to CF individuals who have gating, residual function, splice or conduction mutations [41–44]. It was originally developed for the Gly551Asp-CFTR mutation (G551D; a class III mutation), which results in defective cAMP CFTR channel gating. The gating of the channel reflects the opening and closed states of the CFTR protein. If gating is defective, then a low probability of CFTR channel opening occurs and in turn reduced overall CFTR function. Ivacaftor treatment results in increased chloride transportation across the cell membrane by improving channel gating and thus the time that activated CFTR channels remain open.

The initial phase 3 studies in individuals aged 12 years and older (STRIVE) and those aged between 6 and 12 years of age (ENVISION) evaluated ivacaftor or placebo in patients with at least one Gly551Asp-CFTR mutation. STRIVE identified a significant improvement in percentage predicted (pp) FEV_1 in the treatment arm of 10% at 24 weeks (primary endpoint) that was maintained at 48 weeks. This was together with a 3 kg weight gain, an 8-point increase in the Cystic Fibrosis Questionnaire Revised (CFQ-R) score (an increase in the score out of 100 reflects an improvement in quality of life with a 4-point change being clinically relevant) alongside a reduction in sweat chloride to below the definite diagnostic threshold for CF to a mean of 47.8 mmmol/l [41]. Similar results were demonstrated in children in ENVISION [45]. Participants from both of these studies were then enrolled into the open-labeled extension study (PERSIST) where all individuals received ivacaftor therapy. These individuals maintained the improvements in lung function, weight and exacerbation rates at 144 weeks [46].

5.3 Monotherapy for Phe508del mutations

Such exceptional clinical outcomes were a major advancement in the treatment options for individuals with CF. However, initially modulator therapy was only suitable for approximately 5% of CF individuals as it was only available for gated mutations. Agents that could alter abnormal protein trafficking together with CFTR channel gating and cell membrane surface stability that results from the Phe508del-CFTR mutation (class II mutation) would have a far greater impact upon the CF community. As multiple stages in the CFTR conformational maturation process are affected with the Phe508del-CFTR mutation, different treatment approaches were needed.

HTS therefore progressed to evaluating agents that would be suitable for other mutation classes, focusing on agents could have an impact on dysfunctional protein trafficking [38]. Lumacaftor is an oral corrector agent, which in vitro studies have demonstrated can corrects protein misfolding [47]. However, monotherapy with either ivacaftor or lumacaftor did not lead to clinically relevant improvements in individuals homozygous for the p.Phe508del-CFTR mutation [48, 49].

5.4 Combination therapy: potentiator and corrector agents

As monotherapy only lead to minimal clinically relevant outcomes for Phe508del-homozygotes, the argument strengthened for the use of lumacaftor in combination with ivacaftor. Hence, these two therapies were trialed in combination (Orkambi®). Phase 3 multicentre studies (TRAFFIC and TRANSPORT) of this combination versus placebo elicited a modest gain in absolute pp. FEV_1 of 3% at 24 weeks (primary endpoint) together with significant increases in body mass index (BMI) [50]. The lung function increase being comparatively small to that seen with ivacaftor for gated mutation. However, importantly the 96-week open label extension study (PROGRESS), where all individuals within the initial trials received lumacaftor in combination with ivacaftor, did demonstrate a 42% reduction in the annual rate of lung function decline when compared with matched US registry controls [51]. As rate of lung function decline is known to correlate with morbidity and mortality, this is still a significant outcome [52, 53].

Although lumacaftor in combination with ivacaftor is associated with stabilization of lung disease together with weight improvement, patients can experience various side-effects. Respiratory related adverse events were the commonest complications in the trials and up to 7% of patients discontinued treatment in PROGRESS. In real-world experiences, there have been even higher discontinuation rates of up to 30% [54, 55]. Also, lumacaftor is a potent inducer of the CYP3A4 enzymes and can have interactions with various concurrent medications. Development of other corrector agents with an improved side-effect profile and the potential for enhanced correction of the protein trafficking were therefore required.

This led to the development of tezacaftor, another small molecule corrector agent. Tezacaftor in combination with ivacaftor (Symdeko®/Symveki®), for individuals homozygous for the Phe508del-CFTR mutation, when compared with placebo resulted in a 4% absolute improvement in $ppFEV_1$, together with a five-point improvement in CFQ-R scores but without any significant change in BMI (EVOLVE). Although the increments in lung function were still not as substantial as that seen in ivacaftor use for gating mutations, the adverse events were much lower than with lumacaftor/ivacaftor treatment. The discontinuation rate in the active treatment arm was only 2.9% and none of these were due to respiratory events [56, 57]. It thus appears that the corrector lumacaftor has a poorer side-effect profile than tezacaftor, rather than it being a complete class effect. Tezacaftor/ivacaftor can also be given to patients who have certain residual function and splice mutations (*E56K, P67L, R74W, D110E, D110H, R117C, E193K, L206W, R347H, R352Q, A455E, D579G, 711+3A➔G, E831X, S945L, S977F, F1052V, K1060T, A1067T, R1070W, F1074L, D1152H, D1270N, 2789+5G➔A, 3272-26A➔G, 3849+10kbC➔T*) [58]. Patients with Phe508del and a residual function mutation were studied in the phase III trial EXPAND, which was a crossover study where patients either received tezacaftor-ivacaftor, ivacaftor monotherapy or placebo. The patients were studied for two 8-week intervention periods separated by an 8-week washout period. Change in $ppFEV_1$ (the primary endpoint) was greatest in the treatment arms with a 6.8% increase with tezacaftor-ivacaftor and 4.7% increase with ivacaftor. Both therapies were associated with significant improvements in CFQ-R.

5.5 Future modulator therapy

The combination corrector therapies described, enable individuals with the commonest CF mutation the potential of receiving modulator therapy. However, lumacaftor/ivacaftor and tezacaftor/ivacaftor do not fully restore CFTR protein function. Furthermore, there is still no small molecule therapy for 30% of the individuals with CF who are heterozygotes for Phe508del and have a minimal function (MF) mutation. MF mutations give rise to either the production of defective proteins or no protein production. They include insertion, deletion, nonsense and canonical splice mutations. As up to 90% of CF individuals have one

Phe508del mutation, if small molecule therapy could significantly increase the amount of functional protein for this mutation, a greater range of CF individuals could be treated as then the therapy would be suitable for those individuals with the Phe508del-MF mutations.

Next generation CFTR correctors are under evaluation in combination with tezacaftor/ivacaftor. Phase 2 and 3 trials of these triple therapy agents; VX-659 and VX-445 have provided further exciting results. These corrector agents have a different structure and mechanism of action and provide additive function to the other two agents. For individuals homozygous for Phe508del an increase in absolute $ppFEV_1$ was 9.7% for VX-659 treatment and 11% for VX-445 therapy. Greater increases in lung function were seen for patients with Phe508del-MF mutations; the absolute change in $ppFEV_1$ was 13.3 and 13.8% for VX-659 and VX-445 respectively. These increases were also alongside significant improvements in quality of life and have been maintained in subsequent phase 3 interim report analyses [59–62]. These are incredible outcomes for individuals with more severe mutations and thus who typically have more severe disease phenotypes.

6. Implications of modulator therapy

Important advances in the clinical outcomes for individuals with CF have been possible since the introduction of modulator therapy. Unfortunately these treatments are currently associated with a substantial cost and as a result are not available for all eligible patients. In the United States the Food and Drug Administration (FDA) has approved all four of the currently available modulator therapies. Some European countries and Australia, have access to ivacaftor, lumacaftor/ivacaftor and tezacaftor/ivacaftor [63]. However, worldwide there is significant inequality of access to these agents.

As an increasing number of modulator agents become available, the CF community will need to determine how they can enable patients to receive these expensive therapies. If funding bodies are going to approve them, it is likely that they will require significant clinical outcomes from their use, especially when funding is through a public system.

7. Future directions

The introduction of modulator therapy, particularly when its use becomes widespread, is likely to have an impact upon the range of CF phenotypes. The amount of phenotypic variations should decrease as fewer patients have significant CFTR channel dysfunctional, and it is likely that the disease manifestations will be less severe. It is well known that respiratory related CF disease is associated with less than 10% CFTR channel function and so there is the potential for modulator therapy to have an impact upon this [21]. However, measurements of the degree of change in CFTR channel functionally with the use of modulator therapy is not being undertaken in the clinical setting. The markers being assessed are all surrogate markers of CFTR channel function and include lung function, sweat chloride, weight and quality of life questionnaires. Hence, it will be interesting to see the long-term impact of significant CFTR modulation on the CF cohort when individuals have been on such treatment for many years from birth. Currently a significant improvement is felt to be an increase in $ppFEV_1$ greater than 10%. Time will tell as to whether such changes have a significant impact upon this long-term multi-system disease.

8. Conclusion

The advancements in CF care over the last decade have been remarkable. The use of HTS drug discovery programs have been instrumental in enabling the development of the CFTR modulator agents, first the potentiators and subsequently the corrector agents. The fact that such therapies target the underlying consequence of the CFTR mutation has led to exciting clinical outcomes for individuals with certain CFTR mutations because altering the function of the CFTR protein at the molecular level is essential for true disease change to occur. "Genetic medicines" require a significant improvement in their clinical outcomes before they can become a viable option to modulator therapy. They do however have the advantage that they are not specific for individual mutation classes and could be used as treatment for all patients.

The introduction of newer targeted therapies is transforming CF care, although it remains to be seen how these treatments will impact the CF community in the longer term. Nevertheless, a shift is starting to occur whereby treatments are determined based upon an individual's genetic mutations. It is likely that this will lead to a more personalized model of care and it is hoped a step closer to a cure for this life-limiting disease.

Conflict of interest

CR – no conflict of interest. TK – Clinical Trial Support and Consultancy fees for Vertex Pharmaceuticals, Inc. JW – Clinical Trial Support and Consultancy fees for Vertex Pharmaceuticals, Inc.

Author details

Catherine Rang[1], Tom Kotsimbos[1,2] and John Wilson[1,2*]

1 Department of Respiratory Medicine, Alfred Health, Melbourne, Australia

2 Department of Medicine, Monash University, Melbourne, Australia

*Address all correspondence to: john.wilson@monash.edu

References

[1] The Clinical and Functional Translation of CFTR (CFTR2). Baltimore: Johns Hopkins University. Available from: http://cftr2.org/

[2] Riordan RJ, Kerem B, Alon N, Rozmahel R, Grzelczak Z, et al. Identification of the cystic fibrosis gene: Cloning and characterization of complementary DNA. Science. 1989;**245**(4922):1066-1073

[3] Cystic Fibrosis Foundation Patient Registry. Annual Data Report. Bethesda, Maryland: Cystic Fibrosis Foundation; 2017. p. 2018

[4] Orenti A, Zolin A, Naehrlich L, van Rens J, et al. ECFSPR Annual Report 2016. 2018

[5] Ruseckaite R, Ahern S, Ranger T, Tacey MA, Dean JT, Gardam M, et al. Australian Cystic Fibrosis Data Registry Annual Report 2016. Melbourne, Australia: Monash University, 2018. 45 p

[6] Ratjen F, Bell SC, Rowe SM, Goss CH, Quittner AL, Bush A. Cystic fibrosis. Nature Reviews. Disease Primers. 2015;**1**:15010

[7] Vasiliou V, Vasiliou K, Nebert DW. Human ATP-binding cassette (ABC) transporter family. Human Genomics. 2009;**3**(3):281-290. DOI: 10.1186/1479-7364-3-3-281

[8] Linsdell P. Functional architecture of the CFTR chloride channel. Molecular Membrane Biology. 2014;**31**(1):1-16

[9] Zhang Z, Chen J. Atomic structure of the cystic fibrosis transmembrane conductance regulator. Cell. 2016;**167**(6):1586-1597.e9

[10] Mornon JP, Lehn P, Callebaut I. Molecular models of the open and closed states of the whole human CFTR protein. Cellular and Molecular Life Sciences. 2009;**66**(21):3469-3486

[11] Liu F, Zhang Z, Csanady L, Gadsby DC, Chen J. Molecular structure of the human CFTR ion channel. Cell. 2017;**169**(1):85-95.e8

[12] Kopito RR. Biosynthesis and degradation of CFTR. Physiological Reviews. 1999;**79**(1 Suppl):S167-S173

[13] Riordan JR. Assembly of functional Cftr chloride channels. Annual Review of Physiology. 2005;**67**(1):701-718

[14] Amaral MD. CFTR and chaperones: Processing and degradation. Journal of Molecular Neuroscience. 2004;**23**(1-2):041-048

[15] Farinha CM, Canato S. From the endoplasmic reticulum to the plasma membrane: Mechanisms of CFTR folding and trafficking. Cellular and Molecular Life Sciences. 2017;**74**(1):39-55

[16] Cui L, Aleksandrov L, Chang XB, Hou YX, He L, Hegedus T, et al. Domain interdependence in the biosynthetic assembly of CFTR. Journal of Molecular Biology. 2007;**365**(4):981-994

[17] Atlante A, Favia M, Bobba A, Guerra L, Casavola V, Reshkin SJ. Characterization of mitochondrial function in cells with impaired cystic fibrosis transmembrane conductance regulator (CFTR) function. Journal of Bioenergetics and Biomembranes. 2016;**48**(3):197-210

[18] Ratner D, Mueller C. Immune responses in cystic fibrosis: Are they intrinsically defective? American Journal of Respiratory Cell and Molecular Biology. 2012;**46**(6):715-722

[19] Valdivieso AG, Santa-Coloma TA.CFTR activity and

mitochondrial function. Redox biology. 2013;**1**:190-202

[20] Johnson LG, Olsen JC, Sarkadi B, Moore KL, Swanstrom R, Boucher RC. Efficiency of gene transfer for restoration of normal airway epithelial function in cystic fibrosis. Nature Genetics. 1992;**2**(1):21-25

[21] Alton EW, Boyd AC, Davies JC, Gill DR, Griesenbach U, Harrison PT, et al. Genetic medicines for CF: Hype versus reality. Pediatric Pulmonology. 2016;**51**(S44):S5-S17

[22] Raju SV, Jackson PL, Courville CA, McNicholas CM, Sloane PA, Sabbatini G, et al. Cigarette smoke induces systemic defects in cystic fibrosis transmembrane conductance regulator function. American Journal of Respiratory and Critical Care Medicine. 2013;**188**(11):1321-1330

[23] De Boeck K, Amaral MD. Progress in therapies for cystic fibrosis. The Lancet Respiratory Medicine. 2016;**4**(8):662-674

[24] Ramsey BW, Welsh MJ. AJRCCM: 100-year Anniversary. Progress along the pathway of discovery leading to treatment and cure of cystic fibrosis. American Journal of Respiratory and Critical Care Medicine. 2017;**195**(9):1092-1099

[25] Flotte TR, Laube BL. Gene therapy in cystic fibrosis. Chest. 2001;**120**(3):124S-131S

[26] Gill DR, Hyde SC. Delivery of genes into the CF airway. Thorax. 2014;**69**(10):962-964

[27] Bosch B, De Boeck K. Searching for a cure for cystic fibrosis. A 25-year quest in a nutshell. European Journal of Pediatrics. 2016;**175**(1):1-8

[28] Thaci B, Ulasov IV, Wainwright DA, Lesniak MS. The challenge for gene therapy: Innate immune response to adenoviruses. Oncotarget. 2011;**2**(3):113-121

[29] McLachlan G, Davidson H, Holder E, Davies LA, Pringle IA, Sumner-Jones SG, et al. Pre-clinical evaluation of three non-viral gene transfer agents for cystic fibrosis after aerosol delivery to the ovine lung. Gene Therapy. 2011;**18**(10):996-1005

[30] Alton E, Armstrong DK, Ashby D, Bayfield KJ, Bilton D, Bloomfield EV, et al. Repeated nebulisation of non-viral CFTR gene therapy in patients with cystic fibrosis: A randomised, double-blind, placebo-controlled, phase 2b trial. The Lancet Respiratory Medicine. 2015;**3**(9):684-691

[31] Davies LA, Nunez-Alonso GA, McLachlan G, Hyde SC, Gill DR. Aerosol delivery of DNA/liposomes to the lung for cystic fibrosis gene therapy. Human Gene Therapy. Clinical Development. 2014;**25**(2):97-107

[32] Koehler DR, Frndova H, Leung K, Louca E, Palmer D, Ng P, et al. Aerosol delivery of an enhanced helper-dependent adenovirus formulation to rabbit lung using an intratracheal catheter. The Journal of Gene Medicine. 2005;**7**(11):1409-1420

[33] Haque A, Dewerth A, Antony JS, Riethmuller J, Schweizer GR, Weinmann P, et al. Chemically modified hCFTR mRNAs recuperate lung function in a mouse model of cystic fibrosis. Scientific Reports. 2018;**8**(1):16776

[34] Robinson E, MacDonald KD, Slaughter K, McKinney M, Patel S, Sun C, et al. Lipid nanoparticle-delivered chemically modified mRNA restores chloride secretion in cystic fibrosis. Molecular Therapy. 2018;**26**(8):2034-2046

[35] Zhang JH, Chung TD, Oldenburg KR. A simple statistical parameter for use in evaluation and validation of high throughput screening assays. Journal of Biomolecular Screening. 1999;**4**(2):67-73

[36] González J, Oades K, Leychkis Y, Harootunian A, Negulescu PA. Cell-based assays and instrumentation for screening ion-channel targets. Drug Discovery Today. 1999;**4**(9):431-439

[37] Ma T, Thiagarajah JR, Yang H, Sonawane ND, Folli C, Galietta LJ, et al. Thiazolidinone CFTR inhibitor identified by high-throughput screening blocks cholera toxin-induced intestinal fluid secretion. The Journal of Clinical Investigation. 2002;**110**(11):1651-1658

[38] Van Goor F, Straley KS, Cao D, Gonzalez J, Hadida S, Hazlewood A, et al. Rescue of DeltaF508-CFTR trafficking and gating in human cystic fibrosis airway primary cultures by small molecules. American Journal of Physiology. Lung Cellular and Molecular Physiology. 2006;**290**(6):L1117-L1130

[39] Van Goor F, Hadida S, Grootenhuis PD, Burton B, Cao D, Neuberger T, et al. Rescue of CF airway epithelial cell function in vitro by a CFTR potentiator, VX-770. Proceedings of the National Academy of Sciences of the United States of America. 2009;**106**(44):18825-18830

[40] Sloane PA, Rowe SM. Cystic fibrosis transmembrane conductance regulator protein repair as a therapeutic strategy in cystic fibrosis. Current Opinion in Pulmonary Medicine. 2010;**16**(6):591-597

[41] Ramsey BW, Davies J, McElvaney NG, Tullis E, Bell SC, Drevinek P, et al. A CFTR potentiator in patients with cystic fibrosis and the G551D mutation. The New England Journal of Medicine. 2011;**365**(18):1663-1672

[42] De Boeck K, Munck A, Walker S, Faro A, Hiatt P, Gilmartin G, et al. Efficacy and safety of ivacaftor in patients with cystic fibrosis and a non-G551D gating mutation. Journal of Cystic Fibrosis. 2014;**13**(6):674-680

[43] Van Goor F, Yu H, Burton B, Hoffman BJ. Effect of ivacaftor on CFTR forms with missense mutations associated with defects in protein processing or function. Journal of Cystic Fibrosis. 2014;**13**(1):29-36

[44] Moss RB, Flume PA, Elborn JS, Cooke J, Rowe SM, McColley SA, et al. Efficacy and safety of ivacaftor in patients with cystic fibrosis who have an Arg117His-CFTR mutation: A double-blind, randomised controlled trial. The Lancet Respiratory Medicine. 2015;**3**(7):524-533

[45] Davies JC, Wainwright CE, Canny GJ, Chilvers MA, Howenstine MS, Munck A, et al. Efficacy and safety of ivacaftor in patients aged 6 to 11 years with cystic fibrosis with a G551D mutation. American Journal of Respiratory and Critical Care Medicine. 2013;**187**(11):1219-1225

[46] McKone EF, Borowitz D, Drevinek P, Griese M, Konstan MW, Wainwright C, et al. Long-term safety and efficacy of ivacaftor in patients with cystic fibrosis who have the Gly551Asp- CFTR mutation: A phase 3, open-label extension study (PERSIST). The Lancet Respiratory Medicine. 2014;**2**(11):902-910

[47] Van Goor F, Hadida S, Grootenhuis PD, Burton B, Stack JH, Straley KS, et al. Correction of the F508del-CFTR protein processing defect in vitro by the investigational drug VX-809. Proceedings of the

National Academy of Sciences of the United States of America. 2011;**108**(46):18843-18848

[48] Flume PA, Liou TG, Borowitz DS, Li H, Yen K, Ordonez CL, et al. Ivacaftor in subjects with cystic fibrosis who are homozygous for the F508del-CFTR mutation. Chest. 2012;**142**(3):718-724

[49] Clancy JP, Rowe SM, Accurso FJ, Aitken ML, Amin RS, Ashlock MA, et al. Results of a phase IIa study of VX-809, an investigational CFTR corrector compound, in subjects with cystic fibrosis homozygous for the F508del-CFTR mutation. Thorax. 2012;**67**(1):12-18

[50] Wainwright CE, Elborn JS, Ramsey BW, Marigowda G, Huang X, Cipolli M, et al. Lumacaftor–Ivacaftor in patients with cystic fibrosis homozygous for Phe508del CFTR. New England Journal of Medicine. 2015;**373**(3):220-231

[51] Konstan MW, McKone EF, Moss RB, Marigowda G, Tian S, Waltz D, et al. Assessment of safety and efficacy of long-term treatment with combination lumacaftor and ivacaftor therapy in patients with cystic fibrosis homozygous for the F508del-CFTR mutation (PROGRESS): A phase 3, extension study. The Lancet Respiratory Medicine. 2017;**5**(2):107-118

[52] Kerem E, Reisman J, Corey M, Canny GJ, Levison H. Prediction of mortality in patients with cystic fibrosis. New England Journal of Medicine. 1992;**326**(18):1187-1191

[53] Que C, Cullinan P, Geddes D. Improving rate of decline of FEV1 in young adults with cystic fibrosis. Thorax. 2006;**61**(2):155-157

[54] Jennings MT, Dezube R, Paranjape S, West NE, Hong G, Braun A, et al. An observational study of outcomes and tolerances in patients with cystic fibrosis initiated on lumacaftor/ivacaftor. Annals of the American Thoracic Society. 2017;**14**(11):1662-1666

[55] Hubert D, Chiron R, Camara B, Grenet D, Prevotat A, Bassinet L, et al. Real-life initiation of lumacaftor/ivacaftor combination in adults with cystic fibrosis homozygous for the Phe508del CFTR mutation and severe lung disease. Journal of Cystic Fibrosis. 2017;**16**(3):388-391

[56] Taylor-Cousar JL, Munck A, McKone EF, van der Ent CK, Moeller A, Simard C, et al. Tezacaftor-Ivacaftor in patients with cystic fibrosis homozygous for Phe508del. The New England Journal of Medicine. 2017;**377**(21):2013-2023

[57] Donaldson SH, Pilewski JM, Griese M, Cooke J, Viswanathan L, Tullis E, et al. Tezacaftor/ivacaftor in subjects with cystic fibrosis and F508del/F508del-CFTR or F508del/G551D-CFTR. American Journal of Respiratory and Critical Care Medicine. 2018;**197**(2):214-224

[58] Rowe SM, Daines C, Ringshausen FC, Kerem E, Wilson J, Tullis E, et al. Tezacaftor-ivacaftor in residual-function heterozygotes with cystic fibrosis. The New England Journal of Medicine. 2017;**377**(21):2024-2035

[59] Davies JC, Moskowitz SM, Brown C, Horsley A, Mall MA, McKone EF, et al. VX-659-Tezacaftor-ivacaftor in patients with cystic fibrosis and one or two Phe508del alleles. The New England Journal of Medicine. 2018;**379**(17):1599-1611

[60] Keating D, Marigowda G, Burr L, Daines C, Mall MA, McKone EF, et al. VX-445-Tezacaftor-ivacaftor in patients with cystic fibrosis and one or two Phe508del alleles. The New England Journal of Medicine. 2018;**379**(17):1612-1620

[61] Holguin F. Triple CFTR modulator therapy for cystic fibrosis. The New England Journal of Medicine. 2018;**379**(17):1671-1672

[62] Vertex provides update on ongoing phase 3 program: Two Phase 3 Studies of the Triple Combination of VX-659, Tezacaftor and Ivacaftor Met Primary Endpoint of Improvement in Lung Function (ppFEV1) in People with Cystic Fibrosis Boston; 2018. Available from: https://www.businesswire.com/news/home/20181127005466/en/

[63] Vertex Announces Long-Term Access Agreement in Sweden for Cystic Fibrosis Medicine ORKAMBI® (lumacaftor/ivacaftor). Press release of Vertex Pharamaceuticals London; 2018. Available from: https://www.businesswire.com/news/home/20180618005495/en/

Chapter 4

Evaluating Clinical Effectiveness with CF Registries

Rhonda Szczesniak and Bin Huang

Abstract

Treatment and disease registries have played a vital role in understanding the heterogeneous nature of cystic fibrosis (CF) disease progression. The maturity of so many patient registries and recent national focus on their potential to improve patient-centered outcomes have led to the establishment of guidelines for the conduct of registry data analyses. Despite the insights garnered from utilizing CF patient registries, the analyses are plagued with methodological challenges, such as confounding, missing data, time varying treatment and/or covariates, and treatment-by-selection bias. Nonetheless, these registry studies have been essential for CF clinical effectiveness research. They reflect real-world clinical practice and allow for evaluating patient outcomes in a realistic clinical environment. In this chapter, we reflect on these advancements in registries and study results broadly and specifically in CF. We identify the key statistical challenges with the analysis of CF registry data from start to finish, including design considerations, quality assurance, issues with selection bias, covariate effects, sample size justification and missing data. We describe how these approaches are implemented to answer clinical effectiveness questions and undertake an illustrative example on tobramycin effectiveness and lung function decline.

Keywords: confounding-by-indication bias, instrumental variables, lung function decline, propensity scores, treatment-selection bias

1. Introduction

A registry is "an organized system that uses observational study methods to collect uniform data (clinical or otherwise) to evaluate specified outcomes for a population defined by a particular disease, condition or exposure, and that serves a predetermined scientific, clinical or policy purpose(s)" [1]. Registries and other non-intervention studies are often referred to as *real-world* data to distinguish them from clinical trials or experimental studies.

Treatment and disease registries play a vital role in the advancement of patient-centered outcomes research. These patient registries often include data arising from patient surveillance in observational settings. Numerous epidemiologic studies have used patient registries to characterize disease progression. In more recent years, patient registries have been used for a variety of health-related inquiries, ranging from comparative effectiveness studies to informing clinical decision making at the point of care (see [2], for an example). The maturity of so many patient registries and recent national focuses on their potential to improve patient-centered outcomes have led to the establishment of guidelines for the conduct of registry data analyses [1].

IntechOpen

Although these guidelines are recent, the statistical challenges posed in these observational settings were noted decades ago in epidemiology and public health research [3]. Indeed, registry analyses are plagued with methodological challenges, such as confounding, missing data, time varying treatment and/or covariates, and treatment-by-selection bias.

Despite these challenges, registry studies are essential for clinical effectiveness research. They reflect real-world clinical practice and allow for evaluating patient outcomes in a realistic clinical environment. A registry encompasses the general patient population, including those who are severely ill or less likely to adhere with assigned treatment. These patients commonly are excluded from the randomized controlled trials, and are likely to have very different treatment responses. Further, registry study offers the opportunity to examine important factors such as physician's practice behavior, prescription preference and other covariates pertaining to quality of care, which are impossible to assess in an experimental study. Registry studies commonly include long-term observation and therefore can reflect change of treatment practices, in order to provide a timely assessment of emerging research questions. The use of registry data to evaluate outcomes is of mutual benefit to both patients and clinicians, and it facilitates management of patient care, thereby improving the health care system.

1.1 Evaluating the effectiveness of tobramycin on lung function decline

Throughout the chapter, we will refer to an example from a retrospective longitudinal cohort study, which used the Cystic Fibrosis Foundation Patient Registry (CFFPR) to evaluate the clinical effectiveness of a treatment for lung function decline [4]. Cystic fibrosis (CF) is a lethal autosomal disease in which respiratory failure is the primary cause of death. *Pseudomonas aeruginosa* (*Pa*) is a common, chronic pulmonary infection in CF patients. Inhaled tobramycin (hereafter, Tobi) has been shown to improve lung function in CF patients with Pa in the clinical trial setting. In this example, it is our objective to evaluate the clinical effectiveness—as opposed to efficacy—of Tobi using the CFFPR. We will refer to this case study, in order to illustrate statistical methods for registry data analysis. The Appendix includes analysis implementation using SAS 9.3 (SAS Institute, Cary, NC).

In this chapter, we focus on the design and statistical analyses of patient registry studies. We begin in Section 2 by describing processes to design a study involving registry data, in accordance with the aforementioned guidelines from Gliklich and colleagues. We follow this section with overviews of inferential analyses methods that can be used in registry study to combat selection bias, missing data, time varying treatment or covariates in Section 3. In Section 4, we describe details of the application to the aforementioned patient registry. We discuss the utility of existing methods and remaining analytic challenges in Section 5. Finally, we provide an appendix in Appendix A with implementation of the statistical analyses in our illustrative application.

2. Design considerations for registry studies

Registries may be organized around conditions or exposures (e.g., a cystic fibrosis registry, stroke registry); a healthcare service (e.g., procedure); or a product (drug or device) and can address questions ranging from treatment effectiveness and safety to the quality of care delivered. Registries vary in complexity from simply recording product use as a requirement for reimbursement to more systematic efforts to collect prospective data on many types of treatment, risk factors, and clinical events in a defined population. Follow-up can be retrospective, prospective, or a combination of both. The mode and duration of follow-up can range from days (e.g., hospital admission registry) to decades (e.g., orthopedic implant registry). Constructing and maintaining a large registry requires substantial resources, collaborative effort, and often requires a multi-center or inter-institutional agreement, and a governing body that oversees and coordinates all activities. Typically, there are standard guidelines or written procedures in place that help researchers to gain familiarity and/or access to the registry study.

Before utilizing data from any registry, it is imperative to define the research question and develop a study protocol. Clinical or public health questions of interest should be stated as research questions. Each research question should correspond to a testable hypothesis, which may be assessed using an approach fully described in the statistical considerations (this is particularly important for comparative effectiveness studies).

2.1 Selecting a registry and target population

Finding a registry that is appropriate to answer the research question of interest will require us to review preliminary information about each of the prospective registries, particularly regarding the data elements. For example, consider the following two studies. In each study, it is of interest to determine treatment effectiveness for cystic fibrosis (CF) lung disease. The first study utilized the Cystic Fibrosis Foundation Patient Registry (hereafter, CFFPR) [5] to examine the association between ibuprofen and lung function decline [6, 7]. In a subsequent study, Konstan et al. [8] assessed the relationship between a different treatment, dornase alfa, and lung function decline using registry data from the Epidemiologic Study of Cystic Fibrosis (ESCF) [9]. Although both studies examined treatment effectiveness on the same outcome (lung function decline), each study required distinct data elements to answer the research questions regarding treatment effectiveness. The CFFPR includes data collected on ibuprofen usage; however, the ECSF does not include information for this treatment, eliminating this database as an option for the first study. On the other hand, the ECSF has detailed information on pulmonary symptoms (e.g., coughing), which are known predictors of more rapid lung function decline [7] and therefore need to be considered as potential confounders to assessing treatment effectiveness. Although both registries include data elements to measure dornase alfa usage, which are necessary to answer the research question in the second study, the ECSF enabled the authors to consider detailed pulmonary symptoms as potential confounders. If our research question involves a newly diagnosed condition or rare disorder, we may be limited to a single patient registry. In those instances, the research question may need additional refinement.

In the study protocol, we will need to state the specific objectives. The objective of our CF study is to evaluate the effect of tobramycin on lung function decline. Once the objectives are clarified, we consider the most appropriate study design. In registry analyses, the selection of our study design often depends on how the registry was structured. Registries constructed to capture natural histories are often amenable to studies with longitudinal cohort designs. We can identify the population of interest at this point in the study protocol. Acquiring the subset of data which best reflects the population of interest, exposure variables, and primary and secondary endpoints may include some manipulation of the original registry data files. In our CF example, it is of interest to limit our cohort to individuals chronically infected with *Pseudomonas aeruginosa* (*Pa*). We target this population, since our research question is related to the effectiveness of tobramycin, which is a drug recommended for treating CF chronic *Pa* in patients with CF. In our example, we

Characteristics	Treated with tobramycin	Not treated with tobramycin	P-value[a]
Age, mean ± SD (*n*), y	12.82 ± 4.68 (6451)	12.78 ± 4.59 (6255)	0.84
Male sex, % (*n*)	47.2% (3046)	53.5% (3346)	<0.0001
FEV_1, mean ± SD (*n*), % predicted	74.46 ± 25.33 (6451)	83.69 ± 22.68 (6255)	<0.0001
Weight-for-age percentile, mean ± SD (*n*)	30.05 ± 26.08 (6446)	33.92 ± 26.88 (6252)	<0.0001
CF-related diabetes, % (*n*)	2.3% (150)	1.5% (96)	0.0012
Pancreatic insufficiency, % (*n*)	95.3% (6145)	94.8% (5932)	0.27
No or state/federal insurance, % (*n*)	32.3% (2082)	30.5% (1910)	0.0348
Prior hospitalizations[b]	—	—	—
None, % (*n*)	57.2% (3360)	75.7% (4448)	<0.0001
1, % (*n*)	23.9% (1401)	16.0% (940)	
2, % (*n*)	9.3% (546)	4.6% (273)	
3 or more, % (*n*)	9.6% (566)	3.7% (219)	
Dornase alfa, % (*n*)	79.3% (5116)	49.4% (3087)	<0.0001

Abbreviations: CF, cystic fibrosis; FEV_1, percentage predicted of forced expiratory volume in 1 s.
[a]P-values from Wilcoxon Mann-Whitney or chi-square test.
[b]Number of hospitalizations in the year before baseline.

Table 1.
Descriptive analysis of CF registry variables.

determine chronic *Pa* status for each patient by examining the number of recorded *Pa* infections throughout the calendar year. Our primary endpoint is the mean change in FEV_1% predicted over a 2-year period. We selected additional exposure variables of interest, which are known predictors of change in FEV_1% (see **Table 1**).

2.2 Data elements and quality assurance

For many different types of research, particularly comparative effectiveness research or research involving children and/or rare disease conditions, no single institution has a large enough patient population to perform a proper study. This, along with the growing infrastructures of electronic medical records, has led to an increased effort to create distributed research networks. The widespread adoption of electronic health records (EHRs) has enabled them to become a main source for registry data, capable of capturing the necessary elements as part of routine clinical care, and the ever-changing clinical practices.

The number of data elements and scope of collection often increase over the life of the registry. Well-maintained registries typically include data dictionaries, but verifying data quality specific to our study is essential. In our CF example, we had to calculate specific variables for analysis. Understanding how the data have been collected over time and to what extent (e.g., every clinical encounter) will help determine the appropriate subset of data to extract from the registry. For example, the CFFPR data are collected at every clinical encounter and hospitalization, as well as on an annual basis, on each patient and provided to the CF Foundation. Using descriptive statistics, such as the 5-number summary, mean and standard deviation for each variable, and histograms or boxplots can highlight data discrepancies in continuous variables. Similarly, computing the frequency and percentage of each category in a nominal or ordinal variable may identify variables with questionable entries. Furthermore, summary statistics stratified by calendar year can inform selection of an optimal time frame from natural history registries. In our example, CF-related diabetes, a known predictor of lung function decline that should be included in the analysis, was not collected in earlier calendar years in the CFFPR.

Access to most registries requires approval by a local institutional review board (IRB) prior to data release, and this approval is often necessary to have results of the study peer-reviewed and published. In our experience, developing a protocol that is in accordance with the aforementioned guidelines is sufficient for the IRB review. Although registries rarely contain patient names or medical record numbers, they often include clinical encounter and/or discharge dates. Having this type of protected health information in the data often requires IRB approval.

3. Statistical considerations for comparative effectiveness using registry studies

Statistical analyses in the registry data setting are subject to the statistical challenges previously described for analyses of observational studies [10]. Registries are often established for the purpose of evaluating the effects of interventions. The statistical analysis plan should include appropriate methods to test each hypothesis, methods to address biases and confounding arising from various sources, and sample size/power considerations.

3.1 Selection bias

Regardless of the research question, a registry study will likely be plagued with numerous sources of bias. Selection bias, although inevitable, is typically the most concerning. This type of bias distorts the results for the association of interest and may yield misleading results. Failure to sample from the correct target population and loss to follow-up due to death or some other event are types of selection bias.

A pervasive type of selection bias is confounding by indication, arising from nonrandomized treatment assignment that is often related to the patient's risk to experience poor outcomes. This treatment-by-selection bias creates distinctions between the risk profiles of treated and comparator groups and may violate statistical assumptions in our analyses. In our CF example, treatment selection bias may be more pronounced because the drug in question should only be prescribed to individuals with CF who have a specific chronic infection. Narrowing the cohort to "sicker" individuals can intensify the aforementioned risk profile imbalance between Tobi and non-Tobi groups.

Statistical methods to combat treatment selection bias have been applied in previous studies. Approaches to adjust for treatment selection bias include multivariable regression, propensity score methods, matching and instrumental variables analysis. Stukel et al. [11] applied each of these four approaches to examine the association between cardiac catheterization and long-term acute myocardial infarction mortality. The authors found that the results differed according to the choice of statistical approach. Next, we describe and outline each approach in the context of our CF example.

3.2 Statistical analyses of comparative effectiveness utilized for registry data analysis

3.2.1 Multivariable regression

In the absence of randomization, intervention and comparator groups may exhibit large differences with respect to observed covariates recorded in the registry. This approach, sometimes referred to as covariate adjustment, attempts to account for such differences that may distort estimates of intervention effects (**Figure 1**). Most biomedical studies employ ordinal least squares (OLS) regression to adjust the association between the treatment indicator variable (T_i) and outcome variable (Y) for measured confounders ($X_1, \ldots X_K$). The OLS regression model for each subject ($i = 1, \ldots l$) specifies

$$y_i = \beta_0 + \beta_1 X_1 + \cdots + \beta_K X_K + \gamma T_i + u_i \quad (1)$$

where β_0 is the parameter for the model intercept and μ_i is an error term. Each of the model parameters $\beta_1, \ldots \beta_K$ correspond to the association between the measured confounder and outcome variable. The parameter for treatment effect is γ; we denote its OLS estimate as $\hat{\gamma}$. OLS estimation requires that the error term (u) is not correlated with the measured confounders ($X_1, \ldots X_K$) or the treatment (T). Therefore, the only effect of T on outcome variable (Y) is the direct effect estimated as $\hat{\gamma}$. The challenge of utilizing multivariable regression model for comparative effectiveness is that we must appropriate account for necessary set of confounders. Failure to fully account for necessary confounder may lead to bias estimate of treatment effect.

3.2.2 Propensity score regression

The propensity score (PS) is a summary balancing score indicating the likelihood for a patient to receive the active treatment ($T_i = 1$) using observed set of confounders ($X_1, \ldots X_K$), represented in **Figure 1**. It is a balance score, because by conditioning on the propensity score, one could achieve independence between the treatment assignment and confounders; therefore, propensity scores help to achieve quasi-experiment design for natural occurring treatment assignment in a registry study. The PS can be estimated through a logistic regression modeling

$$logit\, P(T_i = 1) = \beta_0 + \beta_1 X_1 + \cdots + \beta_K X_K \quad (2)$$

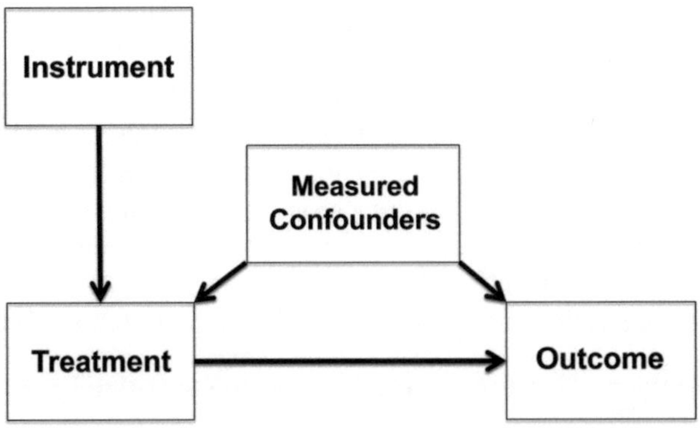

Figure 1.
Causal diagram. The multivariable regression in Model (1) examines the treatment-outcome association, after adjustment for measured confounders. The propensity score methods outlined in Model (2) use the measured confounders to balance the treatment groups (exposure). The IV regression from Model (3) examines the treatment-outcome association, to the extent that the exposure is associated with the instrument. The instrument should not be related the measured confounders; therefore no arrow is drawn for this relationship.

where $logit^{-1}(p) = \log \frac{p}{1-p}$, and the propensity score is estimated by $\hat{\pi}_i = logit^{-1}(\beta_0 + \beta_1 X_1 + \dots + \beta_K X_K)$. There are several propensity score approaches: propensity score adjustment, stratified analyses by the quintiles of propensity score, propensity score sub classification matches treated and untreated patients on their propensity score sub-classes (often by percentiles), and inverse weighting of propensity scores. The first approach includes propensity score directly in the regression equation as a covariate to obtain adjusted treatment effect,

$$y_i = \beta_0 + \beta_1 \pi_1 + \gamma T + u_i \tag{3}$$

The second and the third approaches often categorize patients into five groups using propensity score quintiles. The stratified analyses will perform the regression model of $y_i = \beta_{0,k} + \gamma_k T_i$ for $k = 1, \dots, 5$, and estimate the treatment effect by $\gamma = \sum_{k=1\dots5} \gamma_k / 5$. The PS sub-classification matched analyses will be matching the Tobi and non-Tobi patients on their propensity score groups, then perform analyses for matched pairs. The propensity matching could also be performed on a finer grouping, for example, using 10 groups, or fine matching where a Tobi patient finding matching non-Tobi patient(s) though a distance measure. The method of inverse PS weighting assigns higher (lower) weight to patients who has lower (higher) propensity of receiving Tobi, where the weight is defined as $w_i = \frac{T_i}{ft_i} + \frac{1-T_i}{1-ft_i}$. The intuition behind the weighting approach came from the survey sampling method, and through inverse weighting, one could align the Tobi and non-Tobi patients to have comparable distribution of the confounders. There are advantages and disadvantage of each propensity score methods. Comparisons of these methods can be found in an excellent review paper by Austin and Mandani [12] and the references therein. Different methods are available for deriving propensity score. Other than the logistic regression, one could use more flexible classification and regression tree [13], boosted logistic regression [14], and covariate balancing propensity score method [15]. When applying PS approaches, it is important to check PS balance between the two treatment groups. Patients who have extremely high or low PS values that are not compatible with values from any patients in the other treatment group should be excluded from the PS analyses. The balancing check can be presented in graphic presentation, usually presenting the absolute standardized mean difference (SMD).

3.2.3 Instrumental variables (IV) analysis

One of our primary analysis goals in the registry setting is to identify potential sources of confounding and make the appropriate adjustments in our statistical analysis. Failure to identify sources of measured confounding results in residual confounding. This type of unaddressed confounding goes into the error term, u, which was introduced in Model (1).

Inferential results can also be impacted by what is known as unmeasured confounding. McClellan et al. [16] propose a technique known as instrumental variables (IV) to combat both measured and unmeasured confounding. We introduce the following notation for IV regression. From Model (1), recall that the variables (Y_i, T_i, X_i) correspond to data from the ith patient in the registry, and we assume that there is no correlation between the treatment variable, T_i, and the error term, u_i. This correlation is present when patients receive treatment based on unmeasured characteristics. Let R_i represent an instrument. Consider the following example of a randomized controlled trial. If R_i represents random assignment to treatment, it is the ideal instrument. By construction, it is related to outcome only through treatment assignment [17].

In the typical clinical setting, a provider does not flip a coin to determine whether she will prescribe her patient treatment A, as opposed to some alternative. By construction, *real-world* data contained in registries represent non-random assignment to treatment. Instead, we identify a variable—"an instrument"—that is related to the outcome only through treatment. The variable R_i is a valid instrument, provided the following assumptions are met:

i. R_i is associated with the treatment variable or exposure of interest, T_i;

ii. R_i is not directly associated with the outcome, Y_i; R_i is only associated with Y_i through the treatment variable, T_i

Fortunately, assumption (i) is testable by performing least-squares regression of the proposed IV on the treatment variable and measured confounders:

$$T_i = b_0 + \lambda R_i + b_1 X_1 + \cdots + b_K X_K + \delta_i, \quad (4)$$

where b_0 is the intercept; $b_1, \ldots b_K$ are the parameters corresponding to the aforementioned measured confounders, $X_1, \ldots X_K$; λ is the parameter estimate of the association between the treatment variable, T_i, and the IV, R_i. The magnitude of this association is a measure of the strength of the instrument [17]. Higher magnitude corresponds to greater strength. Let T_i be the resulting prediction of the treatment value, obtained from Model (4). This association is illustrated in **Figure 1** by the arrow moving downward from the instrument to exposure.

We continue this approach, often referred to as two-stage least squares regression, by substituting T_i from Model (4) into the multiple linear regression defined in Model (1):

$$y_i = \beta_0' + \beta_1' X_1 + \cdots + \beta_K' X_K + \gamma' \hat{T}_i + \eta_i \quad (5)$$

In this regression, the same method of estimation is used; however, we use distinct notation because parameter estimates and residual error will differ from Model (1). Finally, we use the estimate of γ' from Model (5) for our interpretations of treatment effect on the outcome. This estimate corresponds to the association in **Figure 1** from treatment to outcome. Note that it is the same path as the multiple linear regression, but the treatment effect has been "instrumented." Assumption (ii) cannot be formally tested, but can be explained in the context of the registry analysis at-hand. We provide this type of explanation in our illustrative application. Sensitivity analyses are imperative to determine the robustness of the IV. We recommend analyzing the data in subgroups to understand how these groups may drive heterogeneous treatment effects.

3.3 Time varying treatment/exposure and covariate

Incorporating time-varying treatment and/or covariate effects is a pervasive issue in registry data analyses. The fundamental challenge arising from the change in treatment and covariates over time often results from a patient's responses and/or experiences with the previous treatment assignment. Thus, simply including the time varying treatment or covariate in such cases could induce bias in estimating treatment effect. Special attention is needed to address this issue when analyzing registry data. Relatively few statistical approaches are available to assess time-varying treatment effects or intermediate outcomes. Hogan and Lancaster [18] proposed inverse probability weighting and instrumental variables as time-varying treatment approaches; another population-based approach is the G-computation formula [19].

3.4 Sample size justification

Completing this process implies that we have carefully considered the hypothesis test and analysis variables, ultimately arriving at a statistical model that will rigorously address the research question. Sample size assessments will differ according to the statistical approach proposed to test the hypothesis, and should incorporate previously established public health or clinical information.

If the statistical approach entails adjustment for confounding and other sources of bias, the sample size calculation is often straightforward. Suppose we plan to test the significance of the treatment effect, γ', previously defined in Model (1), and we have already identified measured confounders (i.e., covariates) that should be included in the model, referred to as $X_1, \cdots X_K$. Our null hypothesis corresponds to $\gamma = 0$, while our alternative hypothesis corresponds to $\gamma \neq 0$. Testing this hypothesis corresponds to determining sample size/power for a multiple linear regression model [20].

We now reconsider the importance of sample size justification for analyses involving a large registry. Statistical significance depends on the sample size and is typically declared if the *P* value obtained from the test statistic falls below a predetermined threshold (e.g., 0.05). This type of significance may be reached in any study, provided that the sample size is large enough; therefore, in addition to this mathematical criterion, we recommend specifying conditions that must be met to achieve practical (public health or clinical) significance within the context of the research question. In biomedical studies, these criteria can often be defined by determining the minimal clinically important difference (MCID). This technique was originally proposed for clinical trials [21] but has spawned several other approaches [22] to determine the MCID. Once we incorporate the MCID into our null and alternative hypothesis statements, we can perform the sample size calculation that corresponds to our proposed inferential analysis.

3.5 Missing data mechanisms and missing data modeling

Missing data can occur in the registry setting for a variety of reasons. Simply put, a missing data point is an observation that should have been recorded; however, for some reason, it was not recorded. It is our desire, as analysts, to understand the reason for this "missingness." In this section, we outline practical analytic approaches to identify potential sources attributable to missing data and methods to combat the resulting bias. We begin with a brief description of the three fundamental missing data mechanisms. For an elegant mathematical treatment of the distinctions among the mechanisms, we refer the reader to the original work by Rubin [23].

3.5.1 Missing completely at random (MCAR)

If the registry data are MCAR, then the reason for missingness is not related to the data that we were able to observe or to the data that we were not able to observe.

We now consider the CF example. MCAR could correspond to the following. The probability of a lung function observation (the outcome variable) being missing from the registry does not depend on any of the observed data (e.g., patient's age) or any of the unobserved data (e.g., having lower lung function does not alter the risk of the observation being missing). Our analysis results from this subset of data will be no different (aside from larger standard errors) than if we had been able to perform the analysis on the entire dataset.

3.5.2 Missing at random (MAR)

This assumption is more relaxed than MCAR but still has specific requirements. For MAR to hold, the missingness cannot be related to unobserved data, given what we have been able to observe. In other words, the missingness can depend upon data that we have already observed (i.e., data entries that were recorded in the registry). Referring again to our CF example, the probability of a lung function observation being missing does not depend upon the actual lung function value, provided that we have the other covariate data. In this case, missingness can depend upon characteristics that have been recorded in the CFFPR (e.g., gender).

3.5.3 Missing not at random (MNAR)

We are more likely to encounter this mechanism in registry data, compared to the other mechanisms. If data are MNAR, then the missingness is related to unobserved data (unlike MAR). The missing observation follows a different distribution than the observed data, regardless of whether the two types of data have other characteristics that are the same. Despite the fact that we have registry data, the data that we are able to observe are not representative of the entire population. Within the CFFPR example, consider the longitudinal data. According to CF Foundation guidelines, patients are supposed to have at least one pulmonary function test per quarter [5]. Suppose there is a subset of patients who do not have lung function data recorded at every clinical encounter. There are many plausible explanations for why these data are missing. For an individual patient, there may be a lack of interest in managing his disease progression, or it could be an entry error. In general, we may lack relations to observed values or those relations may be irrelevant.

In practice, we do not have the information necessary to declare the reason for the missingness. Even thoughtfully developed, well-maintained registries will have missing data; therefore, sensitivity analyses are needed as part of the statistical considerations. As a preliminary step, we recommend creating an indicator (dummy) variable to indicate whether the observation is missing (=1) or otherwise (=0). Regress this dichotomous variable on the other variables to determine whether the missing indicator is associated with observed characteristics. If no association is found, we may conclude that the data are MCAR; however, we still encourage caution when making the MCAR assumption for statistical models using registry data. Although small sample size may produce this result, it is not a likely culprit in settings with large data sources. It is possible that the extent of the missingness may be too low (e.g., 5% of observations are missing) to substantially alter results, but having a low proportion of missing observations is also unlikely in a registry setting. If there is a significant association from our preliminary regression with the indicator variable, then we can rule out the MCAR assumption and more intently investigate the MAR and MNAR assumptions.

We can further examine the MAR assumption by checking for variables that are often missing simultaneously or other potential patterns of missingness. Whenever possible, we recommend performing the analysis under the MAR assumption. The two most common approaches under this mechanism are direct modeling and multiple imputation. Direct modeling implies that we will consider all available data points in our parameter estimation. This method is sometimes referred to as "available case analysis" [24]. In other words, the analysis will not exclude the records of any individual subject who has at least one observed entry. There is a second approach, multiple imputation [25], which has gained favor among analysts with the expansion of computing resources. To perform this approach, several data points for each missing data point are generated, resulting in several distinct dataset. We employ our proposed statistical model separately on each dataset and obtain parameter estimates. The estimates are combined to produce an aggregate estimate. The aggregate estimate and standard error are used to make interpretations of results. This technique is available in many software packages (e.g., SAS proc mi, proc mianalyze).

Unfortunately, there is no way to know whether the data are MAR or MNAR. Previous work by experts in the analysis of missing data has shown that any model we develop under the MNAR assumption will have an equivalent MAR counterpart [26]. Developing an MNAR model requires technical steps that are beyond the scope of our current chapter. Dmitrienko et al. [27] provide an applied approach to investigating MNAR assumptions in the context of sensitivity analyses. Although their text focuses on analyses for data from clinical trials, their approach and accompanying SAS implementation may be adapted to registry data analyses.

3.6 Interpretations of registry data analyses

To simplify interpretation and improve accuracy of the results, sources of potential confounding (measured or unmeasured) should be considered as much in advance as possible. Propensity score regression offers an effective method to further balance the treatment and non-treatment groups. Like multivariable regression, this approach accounts for treatment selection bias [28] only for measured confounders (e.g., measured comorbidities and severity of illness). The propensity score could utilize measured confounders to remove treatment-selection bias. However, when there are unmeasured confounders that determine treatment-selection bias, the propensity-score approach will be limited. In analyzing registry data, IV analyses should be considered when unmeasured confounders are suspected.

Although the IV analysis is a powerful approach, this method has some noteworthy constraints. Large sample size is essential for performing IV analysis, but this issue may not be a challenge in the registry setting. The IV must only affect treatment assignment and have no direct association with outcome. If these assumptions are satisfied, then the IV analysis will yield a consistent estimate of the average causal effect [29]. Assumption (i) is directly testable, but making a heuristic argument for assumption (ii) is a common approach. See Kahn et al. [30] for an example. A weak IV will produce larger standard errors and may lead to incorrect inferential results. This approach is ideal in the presence of small/moderate confounding but becomes less reliable in the presence of large confounding. Admittedly, this is a limitation of the IV analysis in the registry setting. On the other hand, an appropriate IV minimizes the potential impacts of measured and unmeasured confounding [31].

Sensitivity analyses should be performed to examine potential impacts of missing data and particular subgroups that may drive inferential results. Analyses corresponding to the missing at random assumption should be explored in the registry setting. Subgroup analyses are essential to identify heterogeneous treatment effects, particularly in the IV analysis. These sensitivity analyses should be performed regardless of the statistical model that we choose to employ.

4. Illustrative application

4.1 Data summary and descriptive analysis

The CFFPR contains data on individuals receiving care from any CF center in the United States, which has been accredited by the CF Foundation. Like many registries, we underwent an application process to receive the data. The CFFPR data that we received were in separate databases. We used the following two databases. The encounter-level database had one record per patient, per clinical encounter. The annual-level database contained one record per patient, per year. We merged these data to extract the information necessary to determine whether there is a significant association between the use of inhaled tobramycin and lung function in individuals with CF who are chronically infected with *Pa*. Our primary outcome, lung function, was defined as mean change in FEV_1% predicted (FEV_1). In this application, we study short-term effectiveness of inhaled tobramycin, in order to facilitate use of instrumental variables, which still pose several challenges in longitudinal settings with multiple data points and time-varying exposures [17].

We considered the following restrictions to target the study cohort of interest. We requested CFFPR data ranging from January 1, 1998 to December 31, 2009, in order to capture the time at which inhaled tobramycin (Tobi) was recorded in the registry on a consistent basis. We did not consider study records with individuals <6 years of age, due to limitations of modality to measure lung function in young children. We limited the maximum age to 21 years, in an effort to focus on first occurrence of chronic *Pa*. We identified the first chronic Pa infection for each individual by examining all Pa culture results available in the encounter-level data. Patients recorded as having a positive *Pa* culture more than 50% of time in a given year were considered as eligible for the study. This was determined by using the *Pa* culture (indicator) variable available in the CFFPR. We took the first year that the patient had chronic Pa infection as the baseline year. In an effort to keep our study data to one record per patient, we only considered the first chronic *Pa* infection for each patient. Patients who also had another infection at the same time, *Burkholderia cepacia* complex, were not considered as part of the study cohort, because of previously established criteria [32]. An indicator variable for patient-level tobramycin use was defined as receiving inhaled tobramycin within 6 months of initial chronic *Pa*. Baseline FEV_1 was defined as the closest FEV_1 measurement recorded within 6 months after initial chronic *Pa* record. Follow-up FEV_1 was defined as the closest recorded FEV_1 within 1.5–2.5 years of the baseline FEV_1. Patients who did not have a recorded FEV_1 measurement within 6 months after meeting criteria for chronic *Pa* infection were excluded. The outcome variable, decline in FEV_1, was calculated as the difference between follow-up and baseline FEV_1 for each patient. A negative value implies that FEV_1 declined over the 2-year period; a positive value indicates that FEV_1 increased over the 2-year period. **Figure 2** illustrates steps to determining the analysis cohort and resulting sample size.

We identified potential confounders by looking at previous literature (see [6], for example). These variables, measured in the CFFPR, included gender, baseline

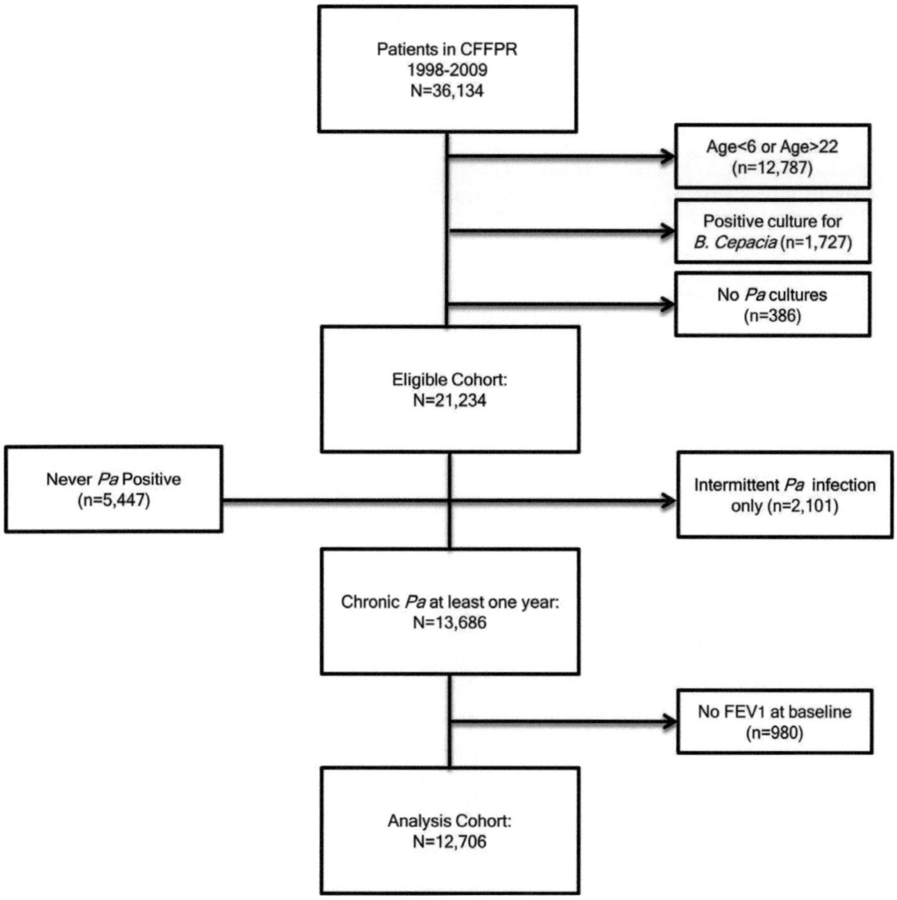

Figure 2.
Diagram of study population in the illustrative CF example, showing inclusion and exclusion steps to obtain an analysis cohort from the registry. CFFPR, Cystic Fibrosis Foundation Patient Registry; Pa, Pseudomonas aeruginosa.

measurements for age, FEV_1, weight-for-age percentile, insurance coverage, CF-related diabetes (with or without fasting hyperglycemia), dornase alfa use, pancreatic insufficiency (defined as taking pancreatic enzymes) and number of hospitalizations in the preceding year. We can compare Tobi and non-Tobi groups with respect to each of these variables using basic inferential testing (i.e., nonparametric test for continuous variables and Chi-square test for categorical variables). Results of the descriptive analysis are presented in **Table 1**. Our descriptive analysis reveals that Tobi and non-Tobi groups differed by several demographic and clinical characteristics. We note that the groups did not differ according to age or being pancreatic insufficient. Next, we utilize the aforementioned statistical models to test this association.

4.2 Multiple linear regression

We use Model (1) to test the association between lung function and tobramycin use, adjusting for potential confounders as covariates, represented as $X_1, \cdots X_K$. **Table 2** shows the results of the multiple linear regression, which suggest that the treated group experienced greater mean decline in $FEV_1\%$ predicted than the

	Type of model	
	Multiple linear regression[a]	Propensity score regression[b]
Covariates	Coefficient (SE), (*P*-value)	Coefficient (SE), (*P*-value)
Patient tobramycin use		
Treated	−1.74 (0.31) (<0.0001)	−1.71 (0.30) (<0.0001)
Not treated	0	0
Age	−0.87 (0.04) (<0.0001)	−0.86 (0.04) (<0.0001)
Baseline FEV_1	−0.27 (0.01) (<0.0001)	−0.27 (0.01) (<0.0001)
Sex		
Female	−1.16 (0.30) (<0.0001)	−1.15 (0.31) (0.0002)
Male	0	0
Weight-for-age percentile	0.06 (0.01) (<0.0001)	0.05 (0.01) (<0.0001)
CF-related diabetes		
Yes	2.06 (1.44) (0.15)	2.19 (1.36) (0.11)
No	0	0
Pancreatic insufficiency	—	—
Yes	0.52 (0.83) (0.54)	0.44 (0.83) (0.60)
No	0	0
Insurance	—	—
None or state/federal	−1.66 (0.34) (<0.0001)	−1.66 (0.34) (<0.0001)
Other	0	0
Baseline hospitalizations[+]	—	—
None	5.05 (0.70) (<0.0001)	4.63 (0.69) (<0.0001)
1	2.74 (0.74)	2.26 (0.74)
2	0.40 (0.87)	0.37 (0.87)
3 or more	0	0
Dornase alfa use	—	—
Yes	−0.46 (0.39) (0.25)	−0.38 (0.40) (0.34)
No	0	0

Abbreviations: CF, cystic fibrosis; FEV_1, percentage predicted of forced expiratory volume in 1 s.
[a]*For each categorical variable in the first-stage model, the coefficient is the difference in patient tobramycin use between the indicated category and the reference category (labeled as coefficient = 0). For each continuous variable, it is the change in patient tobramycin use when the variable is increased by 1 unit. A negative value implies decreased patient tobramycin use.*
[b]*Predicted treatment obtained in Stage 1 serves as propensity score in Stage 2. For each categorical variable in the second-stage model, the coefficient is the difference in FEV_1 decline between the indicated group and the reference group (labeled as coefficient = 0).*
[+]*significant at 2-sided p value < 0.05*
For each continuous variable, it is the change in FEV_1 when the variable is increased by 1 unit. A negative value implies greater FEV_1 decline.

Table 2.
Multiple linear regression and propensity score method to predict lung function decline.

untreated group. Although most covariates were statistically significant at $P < 0.05$, we found that CF-related diabetes, pancreatic insufficiency, and dornase alfa use were not significant predictors of outcome.

4.3 Propensity score method

The patient characteristics at the baseline, which are known to impact FEV outcomes, are considered into the multivariable logistic regression model (Eq. (2)) for estimating propensity scores. **Figure 3** presented the histograms of propensity score for the Tobi treated and not-treated patient groups, showing different but overlapping propensity scores between the two groups. Propensity scores are grouped into five groups by quintiles. The distribution of propensity scores are compared between the Tobi treated and not treated patients within each of the five PS categories; as one could see from **Figure 4**, within each quintile categories, the two patient groups present comparable patterns in their likelihood of receiving

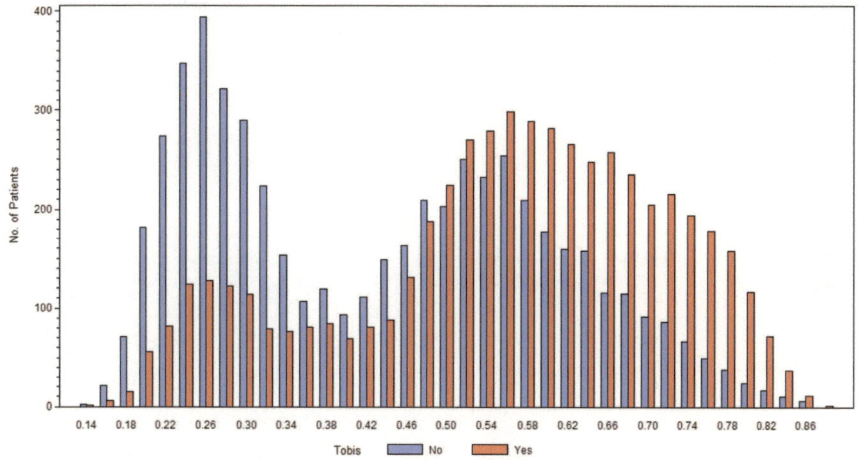

Figure 3.
Histogram of the propensity score distributions by Tobi use (red) and not-group groups (blue). Related the measured confounders; therefore no arrow is drawn for this relationship.

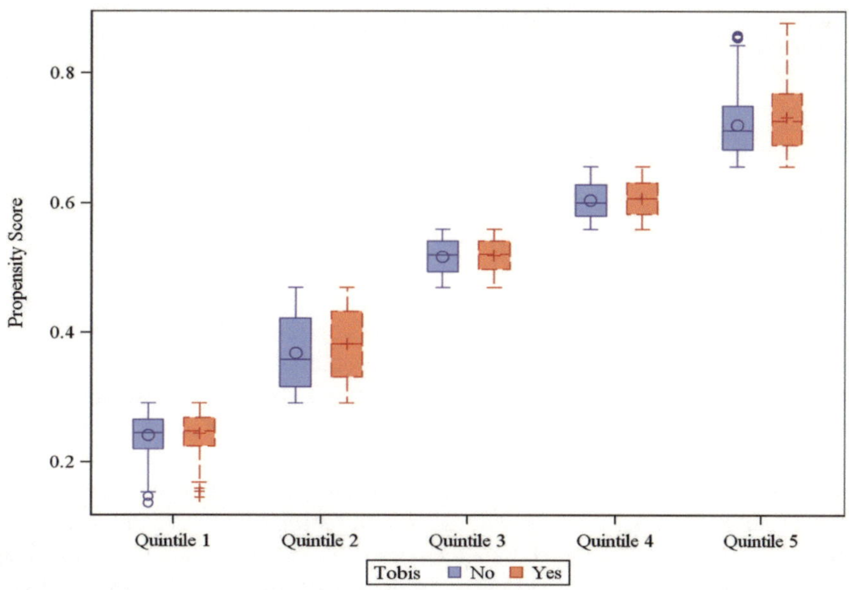

Figure 4.
Box-Whisker plots of the distribution of propensity scores by Tobi use (red) and not use (blue) groups stratified by the quintiles.

Characteristics	Tobi	Level	Before PS matching		After PS matching		After IPW weighting	
			Mean	*P*-value	Mean	*P*-value	Mean	*P*-value
Sex	Treated	Male	47.8%	<0.01	49.1%	0.44	50.8%	0.91
	Not treated		54.0%		48.2%		50.9%	
FEV_1% predicted	Treated		76.38	<0.01	81.68	0.86	81.26	0.85
	Not treated		85.25		81.75		81.17	
Age	Treated		12.10	0.51	11.98	0.73	12.01	0.94
	Not treated		12.05		12.01		12.01	
Weight-for-age percentile	Treated		30.24	<0.01	30.34	0.80	32.33	0.79
	Not treated		33.78		30.18		32.19	
CF-related diabetes	Treated	Yes	1.5%	<0.01	1.3%	0.53	1.2%	0.49
	Not treated		1.0%		1.2%		1.4%	
Pancreatic insufficiency, % (*n*)	Treated	Yes	96.0%	0.94	96.6%	0.85	96.5%	0.72
	Not treated		96.0%		96.7%		96.6%	
No or state/federal insurance	Treated	None or state/federal	30.7%	0.53	30.2%	0.62	30.7%	0.81
	Not treated		30.2%		30.7%		30.5%	
Prior hospitalizations	Treated	None	58.5%	<0.01	69.1%	0.12	67.4%	0.95
		1	23.8%		18.9%		19.8%	
		2	9.4%		6.3%		6.9%	
		3 or more	8.4%		5.7%		5.9%	
	Not treated	None	75.9%		70.2%		67.4%	
		1	16.3%		19.5%		19.7%	
		2	4.6%		5.8%		6.9%	
		3 or more	3.3%		4.6%		6.0%	
Dornase alfa	Treated	Yes	77.6%	<0.01	68.7%	0.24	63.2%	0.88
	Not treated		49.3%		67.4%		63.3%	

Abbreviations: CF, cystic fibrosis; FEV_1, percentage predicted of forced expiratory volume in 1 s; PS, propensity score. Calculations for standardized differences are described in Section 4.3.

Table 3.
Standardized difference (T-val) between Tobi treated and untreated patients.

Tobi. To check for propensity score balance, we compared the Tobi treated and not treated patients on their baseline covariates, the standardized differences between the treated and not treated groups are presented in **Table 3**. The results show that there is a significant difference between the treated and not treated patients groups according to their gender, baseline FEV_1, CF-related diabetes, pancreatic insufficiency, insurance status, prior hospitalization and dornase alfa use. After matching patients on their PS categories, as well as after adjusting by inverse propensity score weighting, we are able to achieve balance between the Tobi treated and not treated groups. Subsequently, we proceed with the propensity score analyses using the inverse propensity score weighted approach. The results are presented in **Table 4**, which can be contrasted with the results from the multivariable regression analyses in **Table 2**. The results from these two approaches are very similar; both are

	Stage 1 (predicts patient tobramycin use)[a]	**Stage 2 (predicts change in lung function)[b]**
Covariates	**Coefficient (SE), (*P*-value)**	**Coefficient (SE), (*P*-value)**
Patient tobramycin use	—	—
Treated	—	2.55 (1.22), (0.0366)
Not treated	—	0
Age	−0.013 (0.003), (0.0002)	−0.86 (0.04), (<0.0001)
Baseline FEV_1	−0.010 (0.001), (<0.0001)	−0.27 (0.01), (<0.0001)
Sex	—	—
Female	0.112 (0.027), (<0.0001)	−1.23 (0.30), (<0.0001)
Male	0	0
Weight-for-age percentile	−0.000 (0.001), (0.74)	0.06 (0.01), (<0.0001)
CF-related diabetes	—	—
Yes	0.112 (1.27), (0.38)	1.93 (1.44), (0.18)
No	0	0
Pancreatic insufficiency	—	—
Yes	0.064 (0.074), (0.39)	0.52 (0.83), (0.54)
No	0	0
Insurance	—	—
None or State/ Federal	−0.128 (0.030), (<0.0001)	−1.58 (0.34), (<0.0001)
Other	0	0
Baseline hospitalizations[+]	—	—
None	−0.598 (0.064), (<0.0001)	5.44 (0.69), (<0.0001)
1	−0.251 (0.068)	2.89 (0.74)
2	−0.148 (0.080)	0.48 (0.87)
3 or more	0	0
Dornase alfa use	—	—
Yes	0.224 (0.036), (<0.0001)	0.28 (0.40), (0.48)
No	0	0

Abbreviations: CF, cystic fibrosis; FEV_1, percentage predicted of forced expiratory volume in 1 s.
**Each model is adjusted for measured confounders by including each listed variable as a covariate. For each categorical variable, the coefficient is the difference in FEV_1 decline between the indicated category and the reference category (labeled as coefficient = 0). For each continuous variable, it is the change in FEV_1 decline when the variable is increased by 1 unit. A negative value implies greater FEV_1 decline.*
[a]Multivariable analysis with standard adjustment for confounding by including characteristics as covariates.
[b]Multivariable analysis weighted using propensity scores.

Table 4.
Instrumental variable analysis to predict lung function decline.*

suggesting negative Tobi treatment effect on the improvement of FEV. The results from randomized clinical trials, however, all suggest a positive Tobi treatment effect. Such differences might be explained by unmeasured confounding that is related to treatment selection bias but not recorded in the registry. We further proceed with IV analyses to examine the Tobi treatment effect.

4.4 Instrumental variables analysis

It is possible that the discrepancy between the previously described registry analysis and clinical trial findings of the treatment effect are due to unmeasured confounding. It is common in observational settings to encounter confounding by indication bias that is not recorded in registries. In this application, we selected a preference-based instrument, center-level prescribing patterns, to combat this bias. The CFFPR includes more than 240 centers. For each center, we calculated the tobramycin-prescribing rate during the time frame of the study. This rate was calculated as the number of times the center prescribed tobramycin to the patient when eligible divided by the total number of times the center should have prescribed tobramycin. We considered a patient to be eligible for the treatment once he met the CFF guidelines for its use.

We had to determine whether the IV met the previously mentioned criteria to be a valid instrument. We began by performing the first-stage analysis outlined in Model (4). We include all potential confounders as explanatory variables, and we include the IV. The response variable in this equation is the tobramycin use. The first-stage results are presented in **Table 4** and reflect what we found in the exploratory analysis from **Table 1**. The IV included in this regression was a highly significant predictor of tobramycin use. The corresponding t-statistic was 28.2, $P < 0.0001$. These results indicate that we have met assumption (i) for center-level prescribing to be a valid instrument. We also note that **Table 4** shows that dornase alfa use is strongly associated with tobramycin use. We will revisit this finding in sensitivity analysis of our instrument. We performed the multiple linear regression specified in Model (5) to determine the association between tobramycin and lung function decline. This regression accounts for observed patient characteristics and provides an instrumented version of tobramycin use. The last column in **Table 4** shows that tobramycin was associated with less FEV_1 decline, suggesting the existence of a positive treatment effect.

Assumption (ii) is not directly testable, but we examine it through sensitivity analyses of heterogeneous treatment effects. These effects may be caused by confounding from other medication use or differences in quality of care received across centers. We performed three different types of sensitivity analyses. First, we extracted quality of care markers through the CF Foundation Annual Report (1) and calculated them for each center. We correlated each marker with our IV and found no significant association. Second, we used subgroup analyses to determine the impact of dornase alfa use on tobramycin effectiveness. We divided the cohort into two distinct groups according to whether they reportedly used dornase alfa. We performed the IV analysis separately on each group. The two sets of results were similar with regard to first- and second-stage analyses. Third, we performed a secondary analysis of patients with *B. cepacia*. Although these patients are traditionally excluded from clinical trials and other effectiveness assessments because of their significantly poorer outcome, they often receive tobramycin in clinical practice. The first-stage analysis of this cohort was similar to the primary results; however, their second-stage analysis showed no significant treatment effect.

4.5 Concluding remarks

Registry data plays an increasingly important role in health care research. Appropriate design and careful statistical approaches to the analyses of registry data are essential. In this chapter, we have described a step-by-step approach to formulating and implementing a registry data analysis. Understanding the research question, selecting the appropriate data source and identifying potential sources of bias are necessary before beginning to construct an analytic plan. The statistical considerations should include data quality assessments and descriptive analyses, and it is critically important to address selection bias due to both measured and unmeasured confounding. This is because selection bias is ubiquitous; failure to adequately address selection bias will lead to biased conclusions. Multivariable regression has been the primary means to combat selection bias. While this technique can help to minimize differences between groups, it is limited to relatively fewer covariates in the adjustment process. Propensity scores, which correspond to the probability of treatment assignment given pre-treatment characteristics, provide a way to summarize multiple covariates into a single score for each individual. Therefore, this approach is capable of handling a large dimension of confounders, which is particularly useful in registry studies when confounders are measured. Another advantage of PS is that it allows one to check between the treatment groups when conditioning on propensity score whether the confounding factors is balanced out. However, when important confounders are not measured, the PS method is limited. One solution is to perform sensitivity analyses by evaluating how estimated treatment effectiveness might change if there exists an unmeasured confounder with varying levels of prevalence. Such practice will allow one to gauge the impact of unmeasured confounders to the treatment effect.

In this example, the likelihood of tobramycin use depends on unmeasured characteristics at the patient, family or care level. The adjustment of unmeasured confounding that is possible through IV analysis may have led to more intuitive conclusions regarding treatment effect. Since CF care is organized by care center, it was reasonable to examine the validity of a preference-based instrument to combat treatment-selection bias. Thorough sensitivity analyses are necessary to examine the robustness of the IV. We limit our illustrative application to a single instrument. It is possible to include multiple instruments and gain more formal properties to testing assumption (ii).

5. Conclusions

When designing and analyzing registry data, it is critically important to address biases and confounding that are inherent in this type of study. Although we have focused, in this chapter, on describing methods for controlling selection biases, registry data are often subject to other types of biases related to measurement and miss-classification error, immortal time bias, loss to follow up, and missing data. We encourage use of sensitivity analyses to understand the impacts of these potential biases to the study conclusions. There are rich literature sources and several guidelines for design and analysis of registry data. In addition to the literature referenced in this chapter, a very useful resource is the recent report on standards in the conduct of registry studies for patient centered outcomes research and the references therein [33].

In addressing selection bias, most often, treatment effects are examined using multiple linear regression with measured confounders included as covariates [34]. Increasingly, PS methods are employed. However, existing statistical methods to address unmeasured confounding may be underutilized in registry settings. The models that we have presented are by no means exhaustive. There is room to develop more methodology, particularly to combat time-varying treatment effects and utilize time-varying instruments [12]. It is possible that preference-based instruments will provide a feasible approach to interrogating registries [14]. Admittedly, there are some situations, such as the IV regression specified in Model (3), where the sample size/power analysis calculation is not straightforward. There are approaches to simulate power for this model, but additional assumptions are necessary. Furthermore, in most controlled studies, we can follow up with subjects who drop out. We rarely have this capability in registry settings, which further limits our ability to diagnose the missing data mechanism.

Acknowledgements

We are grateful to the Cystic Fibrosis Foundation Patient Registry Committee for dispensing the data utilized in the illustrative application. We thank Laurie Kahill, M.S., for information regarding the process of center-specific reporting for this registry. **Tables 1**, **2** and **4** reprinted with permission of the American Thoracic Society.

Conflict of interest

The authors have no relevant conflicts of interest to report.

A. Appendix

Below, we present code from SAS 9.3 (SAS Institute, Cary, NC) to implement the statistical analyses for the application in Section 5.4. See Leslie and Ghomrawi [35] for additional details on the implementation of instrumental variables regression using the QLIM procedure in SAS.

/*For each implementation below, we begin with *analysis_data*, which is the cleaned version of the registry data with all coded variables necessary for analyses. The variable *Tobi* is the indicator variable for whether the subject received tobramycin; *dfev1* refers to the outcome variable (change in FEV_1% predicted). First, we examine the initial difference between the treated and untreated groups.*/

```
title ‘Unadjusted Analysis’;
proc ttest data=analysis_data;
class Tobi;
var dfev1;
run;
```

/*The code below performs a multivariable linear regression to determine the association between tobramycin and change in lung function, with adjustment for the previously described measured confounders. The variables below correspond to sex (*gender*), baseline measures of age (*age*), FEV_1% predicted (*base_fev1*), weight-for-age percentile (*wtpct*), insurance coverage (*inscat*), CF-related diabetes (*cfrd*), dornase alfa (*dnase*), pancreatic insufficiency (*pancr*), and number of hospitalizations in year prior to baseline year (*numhosp*), categorized as 0, 1, 2, 3 or more*/

```
title ‘Model (1): Traditional Regression’;
proc glm data=analysis_data;
class Tobi inscat cfrd dnase pancr numhosp gender;
model dfev1=Tobi base_fev1 wtpct age inscat cfrd dnase pancr numhosp gender/
cl solution;
lsmeans Tobi/pdiff cl;
run;
```

```
/*Next, we implement the propensity score regression model previously
described. First, we use logistic regression to estimate propensity scores for each
subject.*/
title 'Model (2): Propensity Score Regression';
proc logistic data=analysis_data;
class inscat cfrd dnase pancr numhosp gender;
model Tobi=base_fev1 wtpct age inscat cfrd dnase pancr numhosp gender/
link=logit;
output out=props pred=ps;
run;
/*We use the commands below to assign a subject-specific weight that corre-
sponds to his or her propensity score from the logistic regression above. Since the
propensity score, denoted ps below, corresponds to predicted probability of receiv-
ing the treatment, each subject who received the treatment will have weight 1/ps,
while each subject who did not receive the treatment will have weight 1/(1-ps). The
resulting dataset, props2, will consist of the analysis_data, propensity scores that
were previously created and stored in props, and the ps_weight corresponding to
each subject's weighting derived from the propensity score.*/
data props2;
set props;
if Tobi=1 then ps_weight=1/ps;
if Tobi=0 then ps_weight=1/(1-ps);
run;
/*We now implement the weighted multivariable regression. The commands are
similar to our previous regression, except for our use here of the weight statement.
By using this statement, we request computation of weighted means and variance
estimates that are inversely proportional to the corresponding sum of weights.*/
proc glm data=props2;
class Tobi inscat cfrd dnase pancr numhosp gender;
model dfev1=Tobi base_fev1 wtpct age inscat cfrd dnase pancr numhosp gender/
cl solution;
lsmeans Tobi/pdiff cl;
weight ps_weight;
run;
/*Finally, we present commands for the instrumental variables regression. The
first model statement performs the first-stage regression of the treatment indicator
Tobi on the instrument (cid_iv) and all measured confounders. The result is a probit
model with predicted probabilities of tobramycin use for each subject. The second
model statement performs multiple linear regression with the instrumented version
of the tobramycin variable from the first model statement.
title 'Model (3): Instrumental Variables Regression';
proc qlim data=analysis_data;
class inscat cfrd dnase pancr numhosp gender;
model Tobi=cid_iv base_fev1 wtpct age inscat cfrd dnase pancr numhosp gender
/discrete;
model dfev1=base_fev1 wtpct age inscat cfrd dnase pancr numhosp gender /
select(Tobi=1);
output out=Tobi prob proball predicted residual;
run;
```

Author details

Rhonda Szczesniak[1,2]* and Bin Huang[1,2]

1 Division of Biostatistics and Epidemiology, Cincinnati Children's Hospital Medical Center, Cincinnati, Ohio, USA

2 Department of Pediatrics, University of Cincinnati, Cincinnati, Ohio, USA

*Address all correspondence to: rhonda.szczesniak@cchmc.org

References

[1] Gliklich RE, Dreyer NA, editors. Registries for Evaluating Patient Outcomes: A User's Guide. 2nd ed. Rockville, MD: Agency for Healthcare Research and Quality; 2010 (Prepared by Outcome DEcIDE Center [Outcome Sciences, Inc. d/b/a Outcome] under Contract No. HHSA29020050035I TO3); AHRQ Publication No.10-EHC049

[2] McGoon MD, Benza RL, Escribano-Subias P, Jiang X, Miller DP, Peacock AJ, et al. Pulmonary arterial hypertension: Epidemiology and registries. Journal of the American College of Cardiology. 2013;**62**(25 Suppl):D51-D59

[3] Lilienfeld M. Epidemiological methods and inferences in studies of noninfectious diseases PHR review. Public Health Reports. 1957;**72**(1):51-60

[4] VanDyke RD, McPhail GL, Huang B, Fenchel MC, Amin RS, Carle AC, et al. Inhaled tobramycin effectively reduces FEV_1 decline in cystic fibrosis: An instrumental variables analysis. Annals of the American Thoracic Society. 2013; **10**(3):205-212

[5] Cystic Fibrosis Foundation. Patient Registry: 2012 Annual Report; 2013

[6] Konstan MW, Morgan WJ, Butler SM, Pasta DJ, Craib ML, Silva SJ, et al. Risk factors for rate of decline in forced expiratory volume in one second in children and adolescents with cystic fibrosis. The Journal of Pediatrics. 2007; **151**(2):134-139

[7] Konstan MW, Schluchter MD, Xue W, Davis PB. Clinical use of ibuprofen is associated with slower FEV_1 decline in children with cystic fibrosis. American Journal of Respiratory and Critical Care Medicine. 2007;**176**(11):1084-1089

[8] Konstan MW, Wagener JS, Pasta DJ, Millar SJ, Jacobs JR, Yegin A, et al. Clinical use of dornase alfa is associated with a slower rate of FEV_1 decline in cystic fibrosis. Pediatric Pulmonology. 2011;**46**:545-553

[9] Morgan WJ, Butler SM, Johnson CA, Colin AA, Fitzsimmons SC, Geller DE, et al. Epidemiologic study of cystic fibrosis: Design and implementation of a prospective, multicenter, observational study of patients with cystic fibrosis in the U.S. and Canada. Pediatric Pulmonology. 1999;**28**:231-241

[10] Rosenbaum PR. Design of Observational Studies. New York, NY: Springer Series in Statistics; 2009

[11] Stukel TA, Fisher ES, Wennberg DE, Alter DA, Gottlieb DJ, Vermeulen MJ. Analysis of observational studies in the presence of treatment selection bias: Effects of invasive cardiac management on AMI survival using propensity score and instrumental variable methods. JAMA. 2007;**297**(3):278-285

[12] Austin PC, Mamdani MM. A comparison of propensity score methods: A case-study estimating the effectiveness of post-AMI statin use. Statistics in Medicine. 2006;**25**(12): 2084-2106. DOI: 10.1002/sim.2328

[13] Lee BK, Lessler J, Stuart EA. Improving propensity score weighting using machine learning. Statistics in Medicine. 2009;**29**(3):n/a-n/a. DOI: 10.1002/sim.3782

[14] McCaffrey DF, Griffin BA, Almirall D, Slaughter ME, Ramchand R, Burgette LF. A tutorial on propensity score estimation for multiple treatments using generalized boosted models. Statistics in Medicine. 2013;**32**(19):3388-3414. DOI: 10.1002/sim.5753

[15] Imai K, Ratkovic M. Covariate balancing propensity score. Journal of the Royal Statistical Society. Series B:

Statistical Methodology. 2014;**76**(1):243-263. DOI: 10.1111/rssb.12027

[16] McClellan M, McNeil BJ, Newhouse JP. Does more intensive treatment of acute myocardial infarction in the elderly reduce mortality? Analysis using instrumental variables. JAMA. 1994;**272**:859-866

[17] Angrist JD, Imbens GW, Rubin DB. Identification of causal effects using instrumental variables. Journal of the American Statistical Association. 1996;**91**(434):444-455

[18] Hogan JW, Lancaster T. Instrumental variables and inverse probability weighting for causal inference from longitudinal observational studies. Statistical Methods in Medical Research. 2004;**13**:17-48

[19] Robins JM. A new approach to causal inference in mortality studies with a sustained exposure period—Application to control of the healthy worker survivor effect. Mathematical Modeling. 1986;7:1393-1512

[20] Hsieh FY, Bloch DA, Larsen MD. A simple method of sample size calculation for linear and logistic regression. Statistics in Medicine. 1998;**17**:1623-1634

[21] Jaeschke R, Singer J, Guyatt GH. Measurement of health status. Ascertaining the minimal clinically important difference. Controlled Clinical Trials. 1989;**10**(4):407-415

[22] Copay AG, Subach BR, Glassman SD, Polly DW, Schuler TC. Understanding the minimum clinically important difference: A review of concepts and methods. The Spine Journal. 2007;7(5):541-546

[23] Rubin DB. Inference and missing data. Biometrika. 1976;**63**(3):581-592

[24] Kim J-O, Curry J. The treatment of missing data in multivariate analysis. Sociological Methods & Research. 1977;**6**(2):215-240

[25] Schafer JL. Analysis of Incomplete Multivariate Data. London, England: Chapman and Hall; 1997

[26] Molenberghs G, Kenward MG. Missing Data in Clinical Studies. New York, NY: Wiley Statistics in Practice; 2007. p. 286

[27] Dmitrienko A, Molenberghs G, Chuang-Stein C, Offen W. Analysis of Clinical Trials Using SAS®: A Practical Guide. Cary, NC: SAS Institute; 2005. p. 353

[28] Rosenbaum PR, Rubin DB. The central role of the propensity score in observational studies for causal effects. Biometrika. 1983;**70**:41-55

[29] Hernan MA, Robins JM. Instruments for causal inference—An epidemiologist's dream? Epidemiology. 2006;**17**(4):360-372

[30] Kahn KL, Tisnado DM, Adams JL, Liu H, Chen WP, Hu FA, et al. Does ambulatory process of care predict health-related quality of life outcomes for patients with chronic disease? Health Services Research. 2007;**42**:63-83

[31] Newhouse JP, McClellan M. Econometrics in outcomes research: The use of instrumental variables. Annual Review of Public Health. 1998;**19**:17-34

[32] Ramsey BW, Pepe MS, Quan JM, Otto KL, Montgomery AB, Williams-Warren J, et al. Intermittent administration of inhaled tobramycin in patients with cystic fibrosis. The New England Journal of Medicine. 1999;**340**:23-30

[33] PCORI. In: Gliklich RE, Dreyer NA, editors. Standards in the Conduct of Registry Studies for Patient-Centered

Outcomes Research. Methodology Committee, Patient-Centered Outcomes Research Institute (PCORI), by Outcome, A Quintiles Company, PCORI Methodology Standards; 2012. Retrieved from: https://www.pcori.org/sites/default/files/PCORI-Methodology-Standards.pdf

[34] Ionescu-Ittu R, Abrahamowicz M, Pilote L. Treatment effect estimates varied depending on the definition of the provider prescribing preference-based instrumental variables. Journal of Clinical Epidemiology. 2012;**65**:155-162

[35] Leslie RS, Ghomrawi H. The use of propensity scores and instrumental variable methods to adjust for treatment selection bias. SAS Global Forum, Paper 366-2008; 2008

Chapter 5

Liver Changes in the Course of Cystic Fibrosis

Sabina Wiecek

Abstract

Liver damage observed in cystic fibrosis is a complicated process comprised of fibrogenesis, inflammation, remodeling, apoptosis, and cholestasis. Complexity of processes which take place in the liver and bile ducts in the course of this disease are not clearly defined. Changes in the liver are observed in 5–20% of patients with diagnosed cystic fibrosis; however they can increase mortality, shorten time of life, and deteriorate quality of life. The aim of the chapter was to review the risk factors, clinical symptoms, diagnostic methods, and treatment of liver changes in the course of cystic fibrosis.

Keywords: liver, cystic fibrosis

1. Introduction

Hepatic lesions concern only 5–20% of patients with diagnosed cystic fibrosis. However they increase the level of fatalities, shorten the survival rate, and impair the quality of life. Liver diseases are the most common, non-pulmonary cause of death among patients with cystic fibrosis. They most often occur in the first decade of life. Cirrhosis is detected in about 10% of CF children under the age of 18 compared to 2% of adults with the same condition. The average age of the CF liver disease manifestation is about 10 years [1–7].

1.1 Etiopathogenesis of liver's change in patients with cystic fibrosis

Liver and bile duct diseases are a combination of complex processes of fibrosis, inflammation, remodeling, apoptosis, and cholestasis. They are a consequence of the abnormal functioning of the CFTR protein, immunologic reactions, and response to oxidative stress [5, 8–11].

1.1.1 Pathophysiological changes to the bile acids in the course of cystic fibrosis

The important roles played by the pathophysiological changes of the bile duct include changes to the components of the bile (abnormal water and electrolyte contents and change to the pH of the bile) and changes to the profile of bile acids—to hydrophobic, abnormal transport of the bile, retention of toxic bile acids (taurocholic acid), and induction of pro-inflammatory chemokines which influence on biliary fibrogenesis. Factors contributing to the processes of precipitation of bile acids in the bile ducts include decreased synthesis of the salts of the bile acids, decreased absorption of bile acids from the lumen of the small intestine, and

IntechOpen

narrowing of the bile ducts impairing the outflow of the bile from the liver to the lumen of the duodenum [5, 8, 10].

1.1.2 Genetic factors

So far, no specific mutation relating solely to liver damage in the course of cystic fibrosis has been discovered. Most commonly, these are the so-called "serious mutations" of the CFTR gene (delta F508,G524X, N1303K, CFTRdel21kB, 1811 + 1G- > C). The delta F508 mutation plays a particular role in the development of hepatic lesions in the course of cystic fibrosis due to its stimulation of an increased loss of bile acids with stools and the fact that it leads to the formation of more hydrophobic bile acids. Hepatic lesions co- occurring with cystic fibrosis in patients with the 3849 + 10kB C- > T mutation have not yet been the subject of interest. However, the clinical course in patients with diagnosed cystic fibrosis and the same mutation of the CFTR gene tends to vary. There is no strict phenotype–genotype corelation. The role of the SERPINE1 mutation: it occurs in about 2% of the patients with cystic fibrosis and in about 5% of the patients with cystic fibrosis and co-occurring hepatic lesions. Responsible for the synthesis of the inhibitor of serine protease. The protein connected to allele Z is concentrated within the endoplasmic reticulum of hepatocytes leading to their damage, inflammation, and cirrhosis. In about 10% of allele Z homozygotes, the accumulation of the SERPINA gene protein leads to neonatal hepatitis and in 2–3% of cases to fibrosis and cirrhosis. In pathogenesis some genes were suspected as a factor inducing pathological processes in the liver and bile duct in patients with cystic fibrosis (gene of plasminogen activator inhibitor type 1, genes relating to metalloproteinases, P1 glutation s-transferase gene, transforming growth factor beta gene, uridylyltransferase gene (UGT1A1). But the role is not strictly confirmed [12–17].

1.1.3 Immunological factors

Chemokines play a role as an activator of stellate cells (source: hepatic macrophages, endothelial cells, bile duct epithelial cells, lymphocytes, blood platelets, and hepatocytes). The main chemokines are monocyte chemoattractant protein-1 (MCP1), macrophage inflammatory protein-1 beta (MIP1B), TGF-beta, TNF-alpha, platelet-derived growth factor (PDGF), and interleukins IL-1, IL-6, and IL-10 [11, 18–23].

Pathogenesis of hepatic lesions the course of cystic fibrosis according to Colombo [1, 2, 8].

Abnormalities of cholangiocytes.
↓
Mucous plugs in bile ducts.
↓
Inflammatory and proliferative processes.
↓
Focal biliary fibrosis (25–30%).
↓
Multilobular biliary cirrhosis (10%).
↓
Portal hypertension.
↓
Hepatic insufficiency.

1.2 Organ lesions contributing to the manifestation of CFLD

In the examination of Wilchanski et al., the presence of hepatic lesions (cystic fibrosis liver damage (CFLD)) was concluded in 28% (80/288) of CF patients. All patients with hepatic lesions were diagnosed with pancreatic insufficiency. No correlation between the occurrence of hepatic lesions and pulmonary lesions, respiratory insufficiency, the level of malnutrition, meconium ileus, and/or distal intestinal obstruction syndrome (DIOS) was concluded [24]. Lindblad observed meconium ileus in only 12% of CF patients, out of whom only 6/15 patients with meconium ileus had the symptoms of liver damage [6]. Siano did not prove the correlation between the occurrence of hepatic lesions in the course of cystic fibrosis and the pancreatic efficiency and the level of nutrition. In 2–5% of patients, focal biliary cirrhosis develops into multilobular cirrhosis [25].

1.2.1 Nutritional factors

Malnutrition influences on liver function in children with cystic fibrosis. Children with diagnosed cystic fibrosis and liver damage have lower body mass, height, circumference of the upper arm, and BMI. Patients with cystic fibrosis also have significantly lower levels of linoleic (LA), docosahexaenoic (DHA), and docosapentaenoic (DPA) acids. The influence of parenteral nutrition and antioxidant and vitamin deficiency is confirmed [26–29]. Sometimes in children with cystic fibrosis especially with meconium ileus, total parenteral nutrition is necessary. Total parenteral nutrition (TPN) therapy is a well-recognized cause of liver injury. The histologic changes attributed to TPN in the literature vary widely. Total parenteral nutrition-induced liver disease develops in 40–60% of infants who require long-term TPN. The clinical spectrum includes cholestasis, cholelithiasis, hepatic fibrosis with progression to biliary cirrhosis, and the development of portal hypertension and liver failure in a significant number of children who are totally parenterally fed. The pathogenesis is multifactorial and is related to prematurity, low birth weight, and duration of TPN. The degree and severity of the liver disease are related to the recurrent sepsis including catheter sepsis, bacterial translocation, and cholangitis. The lack of enteral feeding leading to reduced gut hormone secretion, reduction of bile flow, and biliary stasis may be important mechanisms in the development of cholestasis, biliary sludge, and cholelithiasis.

1.2.2 The role of medications

In patients with cystic fibrosis, abnormal functions of oxidases and P450, CYP2C8, CYP2C9, and CYP3A4 cytochromes are observed. The dose of beta-lactam should be reduced by 20%. The doses of aminoglycosides should be decided upon depending on the level of the medication in the blood serum. Increased microsomal metabolism relating to theophylline and methylxanthine through the affected first phase of the biotransformation of the medications. Increased hepatic clearance of the second phase, which may be reflected in the abnormal metabolism of furosemide, lorazepam, and ibuprofen [30–32].

1.2.3 Defects of the gall bladder and bile ducts

In about 30% of patients with cystic fibrosis, atrophic gall bladder, or the lack thereof, also its defects and/or of bile ducts is reported. No correlation between cirrhosis and abnormalities in the gall bladder and/or bile ducts has been observed. Gallbladder hydrops and lithiasis are more commonly observed in patients with cystic fibrosis than the healthy population. The narrowing of the distal regions of the bile ducts is frequent and may occur in even 90% of CF patients and contribute to the formation of gallstones [33, 34].

1.2.4 Cholelithiasis

Cholelithiasis concerns 14–24% of CF patients. The following play a role in the pathogenesis of the formation of gallstones: abnormal bile content, increased excretion of bile acids with stools, and the formation of lithogenic bile where bile acids are interlocked with glycine. No correlation between the formation of gallstones and supplementation with pancreatic enzymes has been confirmed [1, 3, 22].

Risk factors for the development of liver diseases in cystic fibrosis:

1. Male gender—three fourths of patients with CFLD are male. Protective role of estrogens in female.

2. Coexisting meconium ileus (inconsistent data—from a five-time higher risk of developing hepatic lesions to a similar risk). Only 25% of patients with CFLD who had meconium ileus in the medical interview was identified. Meconium ileus is not a prerequisite for CFLD. Probably, parenteral nutrition is an additional factor.

3. Significant undernourishment.

4. Pancreatic insufficiency.

5. Severe genotype (delta F508) [1, 12, 24, 35, 36].

1.3 Clinical picture

In most CF patients, the course of hepatic complications is symptomless. Pruritus sometimes occurs and jaundice in patients whose condition is advanced. Incidental finding of hepatomegaly is usually the first sign. In newborns, steatosis may be incidentally discovered in a routine abdominal ultrasound.

Clinical changes of the liver in patients with cystic fibrosis:

1. Focal hepatic fibrosis (72%)

2. Focal biliary cirrhosis (20–30%)

3. Multilobular biliary cirrhosis (5–15%)

4. Portal hypertension (2–5%)

5. Small atrophic gallbladder and narrowing of bile ducts (15–45%)

6. Cholelithiasis (14–24%)

7. Steatosis (25–60%)

8. Cholestasis in newborns (<10%)

9. Primary sclerosing cholangitis (rarely)

10. Cholangiocarcinoma (rarely)

11. Drug-induced, toxic liver damage [1, 3, 12, 24, 37–40]

1.3.1 Laboratory tests

1.3.1.1 Periodic laboratory tests

The levels of AlAT, AspAT, GGTP, bilirubin and bile acids, the APRI index, and FibroTest are recommended. It is believed that elevated levels of at least two hepatic parameters above the norm within at least 3 months is an indication of advancing hepatic lesions. But they have low sensitivity and specificity. Most patients with multifocal cirrhosis have normal test results. Isolated elevation of aminotransferases with concurrent normal GGTP index may indicate steatosis.

1.3.1.2 Abdominal ultrasound with a Doppler option and elastography

Ultrasound is inexpensive and is a noninvasive test. It allows assessment of the level of steatosis, symptoms of portal hypertension, and cirrhotic transformation of the liver. However, normal imaging of the liver does not exclude the ongoing process of fibrosis.

FibroScan is an effective and noninvasive tool to quantify fibrosis and steatosis in the liver diseases including cystic fibrosis. The stiffness of the liver tissue can be assessed based on shear wave velocity (the stiffness increases with the speed).

1.3.1.3 Liver biopsy with histopathological assessment.

Liver biopsy is an invasive procedure and is prone to side effects and sampling. This is not a routine recommended procedure in patients with CFLD.

1.3.1.4 Noninvasive parameters of liver fibrosis

Fibroindex, aminopeptides of type III procollagen, collagen I, collagen IV, laminine, hyaluronic acid, and/or cytokines and chemokines relating to the process of fibrosis. There are studies on their usefulness in minimally invasive clinical diagnostics [27, 41–48].

1.4 Treatment

1. **Background therapy of cystic fibrosis** include pancreas enzyme supplementation, vitamin supplementation, extensive physiotherapy, and nutritional support,

2. **Diet therapy.** In patients with cystic fibrosis, nutrition and survival are intimately related. Growth failure and body mass deficiency are the prognostic factors in patients with CF. Prevention of undernourishment in cystic fibrosis, sometimes feeding tube or PEG nutrition, is recommended. Hypercaloric diet, which is rich in protein, carbohydrates, and fat, is recommended. The energy needs of patients with CF vary widely and have been stated as 120–150% of those required by healthy individuals of the same age, sex, and size. Reduction of protein only in situation of encephalopathy. Correction of fat-soluble vitamin deficiency is essential. Lower serum levels of vitamin A and E were associated with a higher rate of pulmonary exacerbations and worse liver function.

3. **Ursodeoxycholic acid (UDCA).** UDCA has a cytoprotective effect on the cell membranes of cholangiocytes. It stimulates the secretion of chloride ions through calcium-dependent chloride channel. It reduces the ratio of cholic acid in bile (less than 5%), reduces its synthesis, and lowers its overall volume. It also stimulates cholangiocytes and hepatocytes to secrete. It has antiapoptotic effect and reduces the toxic effects of hydrophobic bile acids.

The dose is 15–20 mg/kg b.m. in two divided doses over 24 hours.

There are only a few clinical trials assessing the effectiveness of ursodeoxycholic acid. There is insufficient evidence to justify its routine use in cystic fibrosis as a preventative measure. Present data suggesting that UDCA should be started before severe liver damage is present as it might be able to prevent the progression of CFLD and has the potential to induce a reversal of fibrosis [1, 2, 4, 40, 49–51].

4. The treatment of portal hypertension should include:

- Beta blockers—mild oesophageal varices in patiens without contrindications

- Endoscopic methods for the treatment of severe oesophageal varices [37, 51–53]

5. Liver transplant. Advancing dysfunction of the liver, progressing ascites and jaundice, recurrent bleeding from esophageal varices and hepatopulmonary syndrome, and recurring peritonitis and hepatocarcinoma are indications for liver transplantation. MELD/PELD scores are helpful to evaluate the eligibility for liver transplantation. Model for End-Stage Liver Disease (MELD) includes bilirubin level, albumin, and creatinine concentration. Pediatric end-stage liver disease (PELD) consists of age, bilirubin level, INR index, albumin concentration. PELD/MELD score obtained upon admission may be of help to establish the optimal timing for LT evaluation and listing. A higher score correlates with a more critical condition and worse survival.

In patients with cystic fibrosis following isolated liver transplantation, there is an increased risk of pulmonary complications (severe infections). It seems that an FEV1 < 50% was associated with poor outcomes in isolated liver transplantation, and thus patients with poor lung function should be considered for combined lung-liver transplantation. For isolated liver transplantation, if the FEV1 is <40%, patients are listed with their MELD/PELD score plus a 10% mortality equivalence. If listed for a combined liver-lung transplantation with an FEV1 < 40%, the liver listing starts with a MELD of 40 [54, 55]. Simultaneous liver-pancreas transplantation restores exocrine and endocrine pancreatic function in patients with CFLD and enables improved nutritional outcomes concurrent with the potential for discontinuation of insulin and pancreatic enzyme supplementation therapies. Diabetes has been reported to exert a negative effect on the already decreased pulmonary function, observed in CF patients. FEV1 in CF patients with diabetes is markedly reduced in all age groups compared to CF patients without diabetes. Simultaneous liver-pancreas transplantation is associated with an improved BMI in the post-transplant course [56, 57].

The outcome for combined heart/lung/liver grafting in adult people with CF was poor, whereas liver transplantation alone had acceptable waiting times and good survival outcome. High incidence of renal impairment in this group, and in contrast to previous studies, largely in pediatric patients, respiratory function can decline dramatically [55, 58–61].

European recommendations for the treatment of cystic fibrosis and hepatic lesions:

1. Biochemical tests (AlAT, AspAT, GGTP, FA, prothrombin time, blood platelets) every 6 months.

2. Imaging tests—abdominal ultrasound with Doppler option and elastography, alternatively annual CT or MR.

3. Ursodeoxycholic acid at 20 mg/ g daily with divided doses being more effective.

4. Panendoscopy performed every 2–3 years is necessary in patients with cirrhosis and or splenomegaly in order to exclude esophageal varices.

5. Assessment of the hepatopulmonary syndrome—assessment of intrapulmonary shunts as they intensify hypoxemia.

6. In the case of cirrhosis—assessment of the levels of alpha-fetoprotein (AFP) every 6 months.

7. Mild esophageal varices—nonselective beta blockers? Level 2–3 varices—endoscopic treatment or intrahepatic portosystemic shunts.

8. Prevention of undernutrition (via feeding tube or PEG).

2. Summary

1. The etiopathogenesis of hepatic lesions in the course of cystic fibrosis is very complex and not yet fully explained.

2. The clinical symptoms of CFLD are not characteristic, and the clinical picture is often symptomless or limited.

3. Further studies into the causes of hepatic lesions in cystic fibrosis are necessary, which will contribute to the reduction in the number of deaths, extended survival rate, and improvement in patients' quality of life.

Author details

Sabina Wiecek
Department of Paediatrics, Medical University of Silesia, Katowice, Poland

*Address all correspondence to: sabinawk@wp.pl

References

[1] Colombo C. Liver disease in cystic fibrosis. Current Opinion in Pulmonary Medicine. 2007;**13**:529-536

[2] Colombo C, Alicandro G. Liver disease in cystic fibrosis: Illuminating the black box. Hepatology. 2019 Apr;**69**(4):1379-1381. DOI: 10.1002/hep.30255

[3] Herrmann U, Dockter G, Lammert F. Cystic fibrosis-associated liver disease. Best Practice & Research: Clinical Gastroenterology. 2010;**24**:585-592

[4] Kamal N, Surana P, Koh C. Liver disease in patients with cystic fibrosis. Current Opinion in Gastroenterology. 2018;**34**(3):146-151

[5] Guilbault C, Saeed Z, Downey G, et al. Cystic fibrosis mouse model. American Journal of Respiratory Cell and Molecular Biology. 2007;**36**:1-7

[6] Lindblad A, Glaumann H, Strandvik B. Natural history of liver disease in cystic fibrosis. Hepatology. 1999;**30**(5):1151-1158

[7] Lamireau T, Monnerau S, Martin S, et al. Epidemiology of liver disease in cystic fibrosis: A longitudinal study. Journal of Hepatology. 2004;**41**:920-925

[8] Colombo C, Russo M, Zazzeron L, Romano G. Liver disease in cystic fibrosis. Journal of Pediatric Gastroenterology and Nutrition. 2006;**43**:49-55

[9] Elborn J. Cystic fibrosis. Lancet. 2016;**388**(10059):2519-2531. DOI: 10.1016/S0140-6736(16)00576-6

[10] Fiorotto R, Strazzabosco M. Cystic fibrosis-related liver disease: New paradigm for treatment based on pathophysiology. Clinical Liver Disease. 2016;**8**(5):113-116. DOI: 10.1002/cld.583

[11] Pinzani M, Marra F. Cytokine receptors and signaling in hepatic stellate cells. Seminars in Liver Disease. 2001;**21**:397-416

[12] Bartlett J, Friedmann K, Ling S, et al. Genetic modifiers of liver disease in cystic fibrosis. JAMA. 2009;**9**: 1076-1083

[13] Boëlle PY, Debray D, Guillot L, Corvol H, et al. SERPINA1 Z allele is associated with cystic fibrosis liver disease. Genetics in Medicine. 2019;**21**(9):2151-2155. DOI: 10.1038/s41436-019-0449-6

[14] Debray D, Corvol H, Housset C. Modifier genes in cystic fibrosis-related liver disease. Current Opinion in Gastroenterology. 2019 Mar;**35**(2):88-92. DOI: 10.1097/MOG.0000000000000508

[15] Freudenberg F, Broderick A, Yu B, et al. Pathophysiological basis of liver disease in cystic fibrosis employing a Delta F508 mouse model. American Journal of Physiology-Gastrointestinal and Liver Physiology. 2008;**294**:1411-1420

[16] Fustik S, Traikovska M, Jakovska T, et al. Screening for liver disease in cystic fibrosis: Analysis of clinical and genetic risk factors for its development. The Turkish Journal of Pediatrics. 2008;**50**:526-532

[17] Khan HH, Mew NA, Kaufman SS, et al. Unusual cystic fibrosis transmembrane conductance regulator mutations and liver disease: A case series and review of the literature. Transplantation Proceedings. 2019;**51**(3):790-793. DOI: 10.1016/j

[18] Bergheim I, Guo L, Davis M, et al. Critical role of plasminogen activator inhibitor – 1 in cholestasis liver injury and fibrosis. Journal of Pharmacology

and Experimental Therapeutics. 2006;**316**:592-600

[19] Canbay A, Feldstein A, Baskin-Bey E, et al. The caspase inhibitor IDN-attenuates hepatic injury and fibrosis in the bile duct ligated mouse. The Journal of Pharmacology and Experimental Therapeutics. 2004;**308**(3):1191-1196

[20] Weng H, Ciuclan L, Liu Y, et al. Profibrogenetic transforming growth factor- beta/activin receptor like kinase 5 signaling via connective tissue growth factor expression in hepatocytes. Hepatology. 2007;**46**:1257-1270

[21] Pereira T, Walsh M, Lewindon P, et al. Paediatric cholestatic liver disease: Diagnosis, assessment of disease progression and mechanisms of fibrogenesis. World Journal of Gastrointestinal Pathophysiology. 2010;**15**:69-84

[22] Tanner M, Taylor C. Liver disease in cystic fibrosis. Archives of Disease in Childhood. 1995;**72**:281-284

[23] Tsukamoto H. Cytokine regulation of hepatic stellate cells in liver fibrosis. Alcoholism, Clinical and Experimental Research. 1999;**23**:911-916

[24] Wilschanski M, Rivlin J, Cohen S, et al. Clinical and genetic risk factors for cystic fibrosis – Related liver disease. Pediatrics. 1999;**103**:52-57

[25] Siano M, De Gregorio F, Boggia B, Sepe A, Ferri P, Buonpensiero P, et al. Ursodeoxycholic acid treatment in patients with cystic fibrosis at risk for liver disease. Digestive and Liver Disease. 2010;**42**(6):428-431. DOI: 10.1016/j.dld.2009.07.022

[26] Aldamiz-Echevarria L, Prieto J, Andrade F, et al. Persistence of essential fatty acid deficiency in cystic fibrosis despite nutritional therapy. Pediatric Research. 2009;**66**:585-589

[27] Ayoub F, Trillo-Alvarez C, Morelli G. Risk factors for hepatic steatosis in adults with cystic fibrosis: Similarities to non-alcoholic fatty liver disease. World Journal of Hepatology. 2018;**10**:34-40

[28] Panagopoulou P, Fotoulaki M, Manolitsas A, et al. Adiponectin and body composition in cystic fibrosis. Journal of Cystic Fibrosis. 2008;**7**:244-251

[29] Moriconi N, Kraenzlin M, Muller B, et al. Body composition and adiponectin serum concentration in adult patients with cystic fibrosis. The Journal of Clinical Endocrinology and Metabolism. 2006;**10**:2005-2135

[30] Kearns G. Hepatic drug metabolism in cystic fibrosis: Recent developments and future directions. The Annals of Pharmacotherapy. 1993;**27**:74-79

[31] Rowland M, Gallagher C, O'Laoide R, et al. Outcome in cystic fibrosis liver disease. The American Journal of Gastroenterology. 2011;**106**:104-109

[32] Toledano MB, Mukherjee SK, Howell J, Westaby D, et al. The emerging burden of liver disease in cystic fibrosis patients: A UK nationwide study. PLoS One. 2019;**14**(4):e0212779. DOI: 10.1371/journal.pone.0212779

[33] Curry M, Hegarty J. The gallbladder and biliary tract in cystic fibrosis. Current Gastroenterology Reports. 2005;**7**:147-153

[34] Colombo C, Battezzati P, Crosignani A, et al. Liver disease in cystic fibrosis : A prospective study on incidence, risk factors and outcome. Hepatology. 2002;**36**:1374-1382

[35] De Haan W. A marker associated with increased risk for severe liver disease in cystic fibrosis. Clinical Genetics. 2010;**77**:434-437

[36] Debray D, Narkewicz M, Bodewes F, Colombo C, et al. Cystic fibrosis-related liver disease: Research challenges and future perspectives. Journal of Pediatric Gastroenterology and Nutrition. 2017;**65**(4):443-448. DOI: 10.1097/MPG.0000000000001676

[37] Debray D, Kelly D, Houwen R, et al. Best practice guidance for the diagnosis and management of cystic fibrosis-associated liver disease. Journal of Cystic Fibrosis. 2011;**10**(Suppl. 2):529-536

[38] Potter C, Fishbein M, Hammond S, et al. Can the histologic changes of cystic fibrosis- associated hepatobiliary disease be predicted by clinical criteria? Journal of Pediatric Gastroenterology and Nutrition. 1997;**25**:32-36

[39] Rudnick D. Cystic fibrosis – associated liver disease: When will the future be now? Journal of Pediatric Gastroenterology and Nutrition. 2012;**54**(3):312-317. DOI: 10.1097/MPG.0b013e3182309fd0

[40] Sakiani S, Kleiner DE, Heller T, Koh C. Hepatic manifestations of cystic fibrosis. Clinics in Liver Disease. 2019;**23**(2):263-277. DOI: 10.1016/j.cld.2018.12.008

[41] Aqul A, Jonas M, Harney S, et al. Correlation of transient elastography with severity of cystic fibrosis- related liver disease. Journal of Pediatric Gastroenterology and Nutrition. 2017;**64**:505-511

[42] Alexopoulou A, Pouriki S, Vasilieva L, et al. Evaluation of noninvasive markers for the diagnosis of cystic fibrosis liverdisease. Scandinavian Journal of Gastroenterology. 2018;**53**(12):1547-1552. DOI: 10.1080/00365521.2018.1534986.

[43] Friedrich-Rust M, Schlueter N, Smaczny C, et al. Non-invasive measurement of liver and pancreas fibrosis in patients with cystic fibrosis. Journal of Cystic Fibrosis. 2013;**12**(5):431-439

[44] Leung D, Khan M, Minard C, et al. Aspartate aminotransferase to platelet ratio and fibrosis-4 as biomarkers in biopsy-validated pediatric cystic fibrosis liver disease. Hepatology. 2015;**62**(5):1576-1583

[45] Lewindon PJ, Puertolas-Lopez MV, Ramm LE, et al. Accuracy of transient elastography data combined with APRI in detection and staging of liver disease in pediatric patients with cystic fibrosis. Clinical Gastroenterology and Hepatology. 2019;15. pii: S1542-3565(19)30279-4. DOI: 10.1016/j.cgh.2019.03.015

[46] Loaeza-del-Castillo A, Paz-Pineda F, Oviedo-Cardenas E, et al. AST to platelet ratio index (APRI) for the noninvasive evaluation of liver fibrosis. Annals of Hepatology. 2008;7(4):350-357

[47] Pereira T, Lewindon P, Smith J, et al. Serum markers of hepatic fibrogenesis in cystic fibrosis liver disease. Journal of Hepatology. 2004;**41**:576-583

[48] Sadler M, Crotty P, Fatovich L, et al. Noninvasive methods, including transient elastography, for the detection of liver disease in adults with cystic fibrosis. Canadian Journal of Gastroenterology and Hepatology. 2015;**29**(3):139-144

[49] Lemoine C, Lokar J, McColley S, Alonso E, et al. Cystic fibrosis and portal hypertension: Distal splenorenal shunt can prevent the need for future liver transplant. Journal of Pediatric Surgery. May 2019;**54**(5):1076-1082. DOI: 10.1016/j.jpedsurg.2019.01.035 Epub 2019 Feb 2

[50] Cheng K, Ashby D, Smyth RL. Ursodeoxycholic acid for cystic fibrosis-related liver disease. Cochrane Database of Systematic Reviews.

2017;**9**:CD000222. DOI: 10.1002/14651858.CD000222.pub4.

[51] Pereira T, Lewindon P, Greer R, et al. Transcriptional basis for hepatic fibrosis in cystic fibrosis- associated liver disease. Journal of Pediatric Gastroenterology and Nutrition. 2012;**54**(3):328-335. DOI: 10.1097/MPG.0b013e3182432034

[52] Efrati O, Barak A, Modan-Moses D, et al. Liver cirrhosis and portal hypertension in cystic fibrosis. European Journal of Gastroenterology & Hepatology. 2003;**18**:1073-1078

[53] Stonebraker J, Ooi C, Pace R, et al. Features of severe liver disease with portal hypertension in patients with cystic fibrosis. Clinical Gastroenterology and Hepatology. 2016;**14**(8):1207-1215

[54] Arnon R, Annunzjato R, Miloh T, et al. Liver and combined lung and liver transplantation for cystic fibrosis: Analysis of the UNOS database. Pediatric Transplantation. 2011;**15**:254-264

[55] Freeman AJ, Sellers ZM, MazariegosG,KellyAA.Multidisciplinary approach to pretransplant and posttransplant management of cystic fibrosis-associated liver disease. Liver Transplantation. 2019;**25**(4):640-657. DOI: 10.1002/lt.25421

[56] Frost F, Dyce P, Ochota A, et al. Cystic fibrosis related diabetes: Optimizing care with a multidisciplimaty approach. Diabetes, Metabolic Syndrome and Obesity: Targets and Therapy. 2019;**12**:545-552. DOI: 10.2147/DMSO.S180597

[57] Gan HW, Bhatt JM, Denvir L, et al. Monogenic diabetes mellitus in cystic fibrosis. Archives of Disease in Childhood. 2019;**104**(9):887-889. DOI: 10.1136/archdischild-2018-316141

[58] Arkwright P, Pravica V, Geraghty P, et al. End-organ dysfunction in cystic fibrosis. American Journal of Respiratory and Critical Care Medicine. 2003;**167**:384-389

[59] Bandsma R, Bozic M, Fridell J, et al. Simultaneous liver-pancreas transplantation for cystic fibrosis-related liver disease. A multicenter experience. Journal of Cystic Fibrosis. 2014;**13**:471-477

[60] Nash K, Collier J, French J, et al. Cystic fibrosis liver disease to transplant or not to transplant? American Journal of Transplantation. 2008;**8**:162-169

[61] Young A, Giles C, Mervyn T, et al. A combined liver-pancreas en-bloc transplant in a patient with cystic fibrosis. Transplantation. 2005;**5**:605-607

Chapter 6

Video Call Educational Program for Cystic Fibrosis Adolescents

Annalisa Fogazzi, Fabianna Timelli, Annalisa Vezzoli, Valentina Tradati and Rita Padoan

Abstract

Airway clearance technique (ACT) and inhalation therapy (IT) are essential in cystic fibrosis (CF) lung disease management. We here present our experience with a video-call educational program, which could maintain or improve adherence in adolescents. A 6-month program was offered to adolescents: a physiotherapist would monitor their ACT and IT home program via scheduled video-calls. A structured form evaluating patients' independence and awareness during a session would be filled in at the start and after 6 months. After informed consent was obtained, subjects filled in a questionnaire about their expectations and a satisfaction questionnaire at the end of the program. Student's t-test for paired data was performed for quantitative evaluation of the variables considered in forms filled during video calls. Eleven CF subjects were enrolled; most of them adhered spontaneously, as they expected to improve technique and receive helpful advice. About 301 educational video-calls were performed, 75% being the scheduled calls. Two patients dropped out. In the end, better awareness and self-management in ACT and IT was evident, and patients showed better performances ($P < 0.01$), reporting they received helpful advice. Video-call education is a simple and feasible tool which could be useful to support adherence to ACT and IT in CF adolescents.

Keywords: adherence, patient education, telemedicine

1. Introduction

Adherence to "time-consuming" therapies in chronic patients is a well-recognized issue to overcome.

Low adherence has been described in adolescents suffering from diabetes mellitus [1] and reported in almost 50% of patient prescriptions for respiratory physiotherapy in cystic fibrosis (CF) [2] as well as more recently in prescriptions for drugs targeting cystic fibrosis transmembrane regulator (CFTR) protein function [3].

CF patients from adolescence to adulthood are at risk of their clinical condition worsening, due to several issues: a claim of autonomy (self-management), refusing therapies or parents' authority, and a misunderstanding or low perception of the treatment necessity and efficacy.

It is imperative for CF Centres to ensure awareness, knowledge, and autonomy in adolescents.

A recent review [4] focused on the existing evidence base regarding adherence interventions in adolescents with CF. Among potential strategies to improve adherence, it was suggested to identify social media tools for online support; some preliminary positive experiences have been reported with online educational video. The German Airway League made available video clips about "Correct Inhalation Therapy for Patients with Cystic Fibrosis." This gives the opportunity to CF adolescents to obtain, independently of time and location, autonomously, and in a time-saving manner, information on correct inhalation treatment [5].

An educational video was recently made available to parents of babies who resulted positive at the newborn screening program for cystic fibrosis [6], as an adjunct to help with genetic counseling. This study demonstrated the effectiveness of an educational video in improving parents' knowledge.

We employed a novel face-to-face monitoring of home inhalation therapy (IT) and airway clearance technique (ACT), with a video call survey and educational program, with the aim of assessing awareness of CF adolescents and helping them to improve their knowledge and adherence. Here we present our preliminary experience.

2. Methods and patients

CF adolescents, regularly followed up at our CF Centre, were invited to participate in a 6-month program designed to offer online support during home IT and ACT. All patients in the age range 12–18 years were offered enrollment in the project.

The primary endpoint of the study was the feasibility of the online video call program and its acceptability. Feasibility was determined by percentage of adherence (more than 75% of eligible patients), acceptability by the number of contacts for planned calls (more than 50%), and dropout of enrolled patients (less than 20%).

A secondary endpoint was to assess its efficacy in improving patients' knowledge of therapies (preparation, sequences of IT/ACT) and autonomy in performing respiratory therapies and in cleaning devices, by means of score assigned during video monitoring.

Approval for conducting the study was received by the local ethics committee. Informed consent was obtained from subjects who agreed to participate and from their parents. All patients completed a Q1 questionnaire (see *Appendix*) to investigate their expectations toward the project.

Six touch screen tablets and internet connections were provided to adolescents who did not have access to one.

At the start, all subjects underwent their routine complete functional evaluation (spirometry, 6-minute walking test, MIP/MEP (muscle inspiratory and expiratory pressures)). All have their personalized therapeutic plan (IT and ACT), and during the 6-month program, they received a supervision of their physiotherapy program every 2 months at scheduled clinical visits.

A respiratory physiotherapist, via online video call, monitored, in the early afternoon, the adolescents' home program performances two times a week for 6 months, following each personal therapeutic plan. The scheduled time for each connection was 30–45 minutes; this time was available to monitor both IT and ACT, to answer questions and correct errors.

At the start and end of the study, the physiotherapist filled in a form for each subject, evaluating their independence and awareness during a session. Three issues were assessed, with a total of different items: (a) Does the patient know why, when, and with which drugs to perform IT (3 items)? (b) Does the patient know how to properly prepare the devices (9 items)? (c) Does the patient know to clean and disinfect used devices (2 items)? For each item, a score between 0 and 5 was assigned (0, severely insufficient; 5, excellent). The scores (maximum, sufficient) for each issue were (a) 15, 9; (b) 45, 27; and (c) 10, 6 (see *Appendix*).

With regard to the question "How do you perform ACT?," the physiotherapist, after evaluation of each performance, gave a personalized educational intervention based on deficiencies identified during the video call, giving suggestions and advice and answering questions.

At the end of the study, a Q2 satisfaction questionnaire (see *Appendix*) was filled in by subjects, to evaluate agreement and acceptability of the project and to give their suggestions.

A descriptive analysis of the data collected was performed. A Student's t-test for paired data was performed to assess improvement in scores at the end of the study.

3. Results

Thirty CF patients aged 12–18 years, regularly followed at our CF Centre, were eligible. Participation in the study was offered to all. All but one accepted to participate (97%), and 11 subjects (5 M) on a first arrived basis were enrolled.

The baseline characteristics of the study population are summarized in **Table 1**.

Patients	Sex	Genotype	Respiratory microbiology	Age	FEV_1%	Mip%	Mep %	6′ walking test (m)
1	M	F508 del/ G542X	*Staphylococcus aureus*	13	72	54	58	690
2	M	F508 del/ G542X	*Pseudomonas aeruginosa*	15	51	86	72	720
3	M	1717-1G > A/ N1303K	*Staphylococcus aureus*	13	104	66	63	720
4	F	F508 del/F508 del	*Staphylococcus aureus*	11	94	91	98	605
5	M	F508del/F508 del	*Staphylococcus aureus*	16	69	78	54	591
6	M	F508del/ 1898 + 1GA	*Staphylococcus aureus Pseudomonas aeruginosa*	16	94	108	83	660
7	F	W1282X/ R785X	*Staphylococcus aureus*	11	98	136	114	690
8	F	F508del/ N1303K	*Pseudomonas aeruginosa*	16	69	151	149	570
9	F	F508 del/F508 del	*Non-tuberculous Mycobacterium*	16	56	128	87	Not done
10	F	F508del/ G673X	*Achromobacter xyl. Staphylococcus aureus*	13	61	167	95	557
11	F	F508del/ W1282X	*Staphylococcus aureus*	12	79	118	96	695
Mean				**13.82**	**77.00**	**107.55**	**88.09**	**649.80**
SD				**2.04**	**18.11**	**36.01**	**27.52**	**62.96**

Table 1.
Clinical characteristics of the study population at the baseline visit.

All subjects have a confirmed CF, and all presented pancreatic insufficiency, age ranged between 11 and 16 years. Seven subjects had moderate respiratory disease (FEV_1pp: 51–79%); four had normal function (FEV_1pp: 94–104%). Chronic *Pseudomonas* infection was present in three. All presented a 6-minute walking test within the normal limits (range 557–720 meters).

Airway clearance technique consisted of the use of PEP Mask in all of them.

In the 6-month program, 301 educational video calls were performed, which is 75% of the scheduled calls.

Their mean duration was 45 min (range 30–60 min). Each subject received a video call at least twice a week.

During the study period, two subjects dropped out (n°9 and 10; 18%), because of school commitments in the afternoon.

Regarding questionnaires filled in by subjects at the start (Q1) and at the end (Q2) of the project, Q1 (filled by 11 subjects) shows that eight adolescents were pleased to participate in the project, considering it an opportunity to maintain frequent contact with physiotherapists (in four cases) and a way to monitor their home program (in five). Nine subjects adhered spontaneously, but four did it for pleasing parents, and only one boy was forced by them. All subjects considered ACT very important to maintain their health, and their main expectations were to improve technique and receive helpful advice (six subjects) and have the opportunity to demonstrate their independence (two of them).

The Q2 questionnaire (filled in by nine subjects) shows that ACT was considered important in spite of the effort it requires. All of them were pleased to be enrolled in the study as it was a good opportunity to monitor the way they perform ACT; they have received helpful advice (reported by five of them) or have maintained contact with physiotherapists (by four). Four of them felt emotionally supported.

3.1 Results from forms filled by the physiotherapist

Issue A. *Does the subject know why, when, and with which drugs to perform IT and ACT* (possible score for each patient: 0–15)? At the start, 4 out of 11 adolescents did not know the reason for which they must perform the IT/ACT, and they did not perform both the IT and the ACT correctly. At the end, the final scores showed a greater awareness of why airway clearance is important and have shown a better understanding of IT in all subjects but one (mean score at start 6.5 (range 2–13), mean score at end 9.6 (range 5–14), ($P < 0.01$)).

Issue B. *Does the subject properly prepare his/her IT and device* (possible score for each patient: 0–45)? At the first evaluation, almost all were already able to prepare and assemble the devices; at the final one, all subjects were able to prepare and assemble the devices (mean score at start 29.5 (range 13–43), mean score at end 35.8 (range 25–43), ($P < 0.01$)).

Issue C. *Does the subject clean and disinfect his/her devices after therapy* (possible score 0–10)? None but one subject was autonomous in device cleaning and disinfection, leaving this duty to parents, both at the start and end (mean score 2.2 in both evaluations, NS).

The initial assessment of appropriateness in the execution of IT/ACT shows that seven subjects kept a right posture during IT/ACT and respected the correct sequence of drugs, but after the educational intervention, all of them performed the entire sequence IT / ACT appropriately.

4. Discussion

Our preliminary experience on a limited number of CF adolescents shows the possibility to perform an educational program by means of online video call. This program was designed to offer online support during home IT and ACT by a respiratory physiotherapist, with the aim of improving knowledge and adherence to respiratory physiotherapy in CF adolescents.

Recent reported experiences on an educational program on inhalation therapy [5] or newborn screening [6] with online video clips do not provide any kind of personal relationship between those who produced the media available online and the CF patient, differently by our program.

New technologies such as video call using smartphones or tablets are used on a daily basis by adolescents; thus we hypothesized that introducing educational programs in their life using these technologies might result in better outcomes. To the best of our knowledge, our study is the first educational program to use online video calls provided by an experienced physiotherapist to monitor IT/ACT. This program gave the opportunity to CF teenagers to develop personal contact with the respiratory therapist in their own homes, beyond the scheduled visits at the specialist center. Our work proved the feasibility of an educational video call program, where adolescents accepted online supervision for their daily IT/ACT and attended 75% of the planned calls.

The main problem we faced was the timing of the video calls, scheduled in the afternoon. In fact, 2 out of 11 patients had to abandon the project because of the video call time coinciding with commitments to school.

ACT monitoring and individualized educational interventions in the short term seem to lead to positive results, such as increased knowledge and better adherence to prescribed therapies by the end of the project.

Patients agreed to receive video calls and maintain frequent contact with the physiotherapist, and the program seemed to improve their autonomy in the management of IT and ACT.

With this study, we have also verified how an aspect of daily care, cleaning, and disinfection of IT/ACT devices is not taken into account as a personal task by teenagers but is constantly referred to one of the parents (usually the mother). An explanation could be also the desire of parents to be sure of the adequacy of cleaning or to be still present in the care of their teenage children.

Since the acquisition of personal autonomy also involves care (cleaning and disinfection) of the tools necessary for the execution of airway clearance, we will implement educational programs on this aspect of care.

The main positive effects of this project were the CF care team showed both the willingness and capability of using modern technologies to communicate with young people and improvement in knowledge, self-management, and autonomy in CF patients.

After the study ended, as a result of the project and in response to our patients' requests, video calls were made available during intravenous home therapy for pulmonary exacerbations, as patients recognized its usefulness in improving adherence.

Making additional resources available to patients outside the CF clinics, at their own home, resulted to be beneficial in reducing the feeling of loneliness during ACT daily performance and may, therefore, promote motivation and ameliorate adherence.

This pilot study has some limitations, including the low number of patients and its short duration. It is well known that educational interventions must be repeated in time, with scheduled follow-up calls to maintain their efficacy. However, the primary outcome was to test the feasibility of an educational program via video calls, and this has been achieved, thanks to a rethinking of the CF health services model, which was delivered to patients' homes via online video calls.

The bias of the study is the very small number of patients.

In the future, further studies are needed to explore feasibility/acceptability with a larger number of subjects and clarify the duration needed to maintain positive results in the long term and its usefulness during home therapy for pulmonary exacerbations.

In conclusion, our pilot experience verified the feasibility and acceptability of an online video call educational program designed to improve knowledge and self-management of CF adolescents.

ACT monitoring and educational interventions, performed by video call, significantly improved our patients' ability and knowledge, promoting their adherence to ACT/IT and awareness of the need for greater adherence to the therapeutic program. Their independence has also been promoted. Video call educational programs could be a helpful therapeutic tool in the CF scenario.

4.1 Psychological comment

The design of this study also arises from the deep consideration of the psychological aspects related to the adolescent world of our age and in particular to the portion of the adolescent world that must live with a chronic disease caused by the presence of cystic fibrosis.

This is particularly true and relevant in a perspective that strongly supports the goodness and efficacy of the treatment being facilitated by the personalization of the therapeutic plan, modulated according to the characteristics and specific resources of the patient it is addressed to.

The current adolescent generation is embodied by the so-called "digital natives," namely, children and teenagers who have grown up hand in hand with the increasingly intensive use of the Internet, in an age where the use of technology breaks deep into everyday life, with a dramatic surge in virtual relationships that change and significantly influence the profile of contemporary adolescents.

Adolescence is a complex age with difficult specific-phase tasks to perform, even more so for the chronically ill adolescent, whose emotional world is permeated by difficult balances.

Girls and boys dealing with the disease are progressively confronted with aspects of themselves and of their pathology that binds them to a condition of dependence and fragility. This condition acquires anti-evolutionary meaning, in stark contrast with the increasing search for emancipation, autonomy, and self-affirmation.

Parents, in turn, are mainly concerned about their children's health and survival and often tend to limit their autonomy, with an excessive overprotection and control over the care and daily life of their children, thus possibly producing results that are quite opposite to their expectations, i.e., poor adherence to the prescribed therapy and onset of risk behaviors.

Therefore, respiratory physiotherapy represents an extremely delicate and meaningful moment for adolescents with cystic fibrosis, as it is a constant reminder of their chronic condition: they are chronically ill individuals who depend on a treatment they would most like to avoid. Physiotherapy inevitably turns into a battlefield where parents and children fight every day, causing distress and strain on both sides.

In light of these considerations, the project aiming at promoting the improvement of physiotherapy through video calls is even more relevant because it pursues multiple objectives.

On the one hand, it allows a personalized educational intervention aimed at supporting the improvement of techniques and skills by adolescent patients, taking advantage of technology and the Internet, which directly provide a familiar common language, appreciated by the youth and able to abolish distance.

On the other hand, the operator has the opportunity to walk into the homes of children and parents, albeit virtually, reducing the sense of loneliness and supporting the fatigue that adhering to such demanding regimens involves, especially during adolescence, thus encouraging a gradual autonomy, which is a fundamental objective both for the treatment and for the adherence to the therapies as well as for the growth and for the psychological well-being of our patients.

Acknowledgements

This study was supported thanks to a Grant from GILEAD (Gilead Award 2014). We are grateful to Francesco Fiorini, MD for his linguist revision of the manuscript.

A. Appendix

1. Questionnaire #1

2. Video Call Educational Program (Evaluation Form)

3. Questionnaire #2

A.1 Questionnaire # 1

Dear boys and girls, we ask you to fill this questionnaire before the beginning of the study.

The aim is to understand your expectation about this project. The questionnaire is anonymous; fill only your age and gender.

Thanks for your collaboration.

Dr. Padoan and Physiotherapists.

1. Are you happy to be involved in this study?

o Yes

o No

o Indifferent

1a. If you answered "yes," please explain why:

o It is a way to monitor my physiotherapy.

o I like the technology.

o I am happy to receive support in my home treatment.

- I like the idea to receive support by the physiotherapist.
- I want to receive a tablet.
- I think that this project improves my adherence to the treatment.
- Other, please explain...

1b. If you answered "no," please explain why:

- Hospital visits are enough, I do not want to be checked at home.
- These scheduled calls limit my freedom.
- I do not like using computer.
- I think to do physiotherapy correctly so I do not need help.
- I think that physiotherapy is not such important for my health.
- Other, please explain..

1c. If you answered "indifferent," explain why:

- I do not know if this project could be useful for me.
- I do not understand what the project consists in.
- Other, please explain..

2. I have agreed to participate in the project:

- Deciding by myself without any advice.
- Because my parents forced me.
- I decide alone with the awareness that this choice is the best for my parents.

3. To maintain your health, do you think that physiotherapy is:

- Very important.
- Not so important.
- Not important at all.
- I know that it's very important for my health but I do not want to perform it.
- Other, please explain..

4. Why do physician and physiotherapists involve you in this project? What do you think?

- ○ Because they do not believe that I perform my daily physiotherapy
- ○ Because they believe that I do not correctly perform it
- ○ Because they want to help me to feel good
- ○ Because they want to control me
- ○ To make my parents happy
- ○ To help me to become autonomous and responsible for my therapy

5. What do you expect from this project?

- ○ Being able to perform physiotherapy better than before.
- ○ To receive advice and useful information.
- ○ To receive support during my therapy.
- ○ To prove that I am able to do things well.
- ○ To please my parents, so that they "stress" me less for physiotherapy.
- ○ To feel supported even emotionally.
- ○ To waste time that I could use to do something else.
- ○ To "earn" a tablet.
- ○ I do not expect anything in particular.
- ○ Other, please explain...

6. Do you want to tell us something else?

....

Your age ....
You are

- ○ Male
- ○ Female

A.2 Video Call Educational Program (Evaluation Form)

Evaluation Date:.................
Patient's first and last name: ....
Sex of the patient: ♂ Male ♀ Female Age of the patient ....years.
The following assessment is:

- ○ *Initial*
- ○ *Intermediate (3 months)*
- ○ *Final*

A. Knowledge of therapy

	0	1	2	3	4	5
1. Does the patient know why he/she had to do respiratory physiotherapy?						
2. Does the patient know the correct sequence of respiratory physiotherapy (nasal lavage-bronchodilators-hypertonic/Pulmozyme/mucolytic-physiotherapy-antibiotic therapy)?						
3. Does the patient know the drugs he/she takes by aerosol (short-acting bronchodilators, bronchodilators and long-acting corticosteroids, oral steroids, antibiotics, Pulmozyme/hypertonic/mucolytic, etc.)?						

Legend:
5 = Excellent; 4 = Good; 3 = Discrete; 2 = Sufficient; 1 = Insufficient; 0 = Severely insufficient.

Educational notes (e.g., acknowledgment of need for education in a given area or on a specific aspect, etc.):

....
....
....
....

B. Execution of respiratory physiotherapy session

	0	1	2	3	4	5
1. Is the patient able to prepare the necessary material for the execution of the physiotherapy session (Lavonase, compressor, nebulizer ampoule, PEP Mask, or other devices)?						
2. Is the material clean and in good condition before the session?						
3. When performing the aerosol, does the patient choose the correct interface?						
4. If the patient uses the PEP Mask, is he/she able to fit the various components (mask, resistor, valve) in the correct way?						
5. If the patient uses the PEP Mask, does he/she employ the correct resistor?						
6. Does the patient respect the correct timing during the airway clearance technique?						
7. Does the patient perform FET or cough?						
8. Is the patient able to produce sputum?						
9. Is the patient's posture correct during the session of respiratory physiotherapy?						

Legend:
5 = Excellent; 4 = Good; 3 = Discrete; 2 = Sufficient; 1 = Insufficient; 0 = Severely insufficient.

Educational notes (e.g., acknowledgment of need for education in a given area or on a specific aspect, etc.):

....

....

....

....

....

C. Cleaning devices

	0	1	2	3	4	5
1. Does the patient clean the devices?						
2. Does the patient disinfect the devices?						

Legend:
5 = Excellent; 4 = Good; 3 = Discrete; 2 = Sufficient; 1 = Insufficient; 0 = Severely insufficient.

Educational notes (e.g., acknowledgment of need for education in a given area or on a specific aspect, etc.):

....

....

....

....

....

Signature of the physiotherapist.

....

A.3 Questionnaire #2

Dear boys and girls, this short questionnaire follows the project "Monitoring of Respiratory Physiotherapy Through Video Call in Adolescents." The aim is to know what you think about the project and its utility and receive suggestion from you.

The questionnaire is anonymous; fill only your age and gender.

Thanks for your collaboration!

Dr. Padoan and physiotherapist.

1. Are you happy to have been involved in this project?

- Yes
- No
- Indifferent

1a. If you answered "yes," please explain why:

- It was a way to monitor my physiotherapy.
- I love the technology.

- I was happy to receive support in my home treatment.
- I liked the idea to receive support by the physiotherapist.
- I wanted to receive a tablet.
- I thought that this project would improve my adherence to the treatment.
- Other, please explain.

1b. If you answered "no," please explain why:

- Hospital visits were enough, I did not want to be checked at home.
- These scheduled calls limited my freedom.
- I do not like using computer.
- I thought to perform physiotherapy correctly so I did not need help.
- I thought that physiotherapy is not such important for my health.
- Other, please explain...
....

1c. If you answered "indifferent," please explain why:
....
....

2. What do you think about your respiratory physiotherapy?

- It is very important.
- It is not so important.
- It is not important at all.
- It is very important to feel better but I do not want to perform it.
- Other, please explain...
....

3. What do you think about your involvement in this project by the physiotherapist?

- Physiotherapists did not believe that I perform my daily physiotherapy.
- Physiotherapists believed I do not perform correctly my daily physiotherapy.
- Physiotherapists wanted to make me feel better.
- Physiotherapists wanted to control me.

- ○ Physiotherapists wanted to make my parents happy.
- ○ Physiotherapists wanted to help me to become autonomous and responsible for my therapy.

4. What do you think at the end of this project?

- ○ I'm able to better perform physiotherapy.
- ○ I received advice and useful information.
- ○ I proved my ability to perform physiotherapy.
- ○ I pleased my parents.
- ○ I felt supported even emotionally.
- ○ I wasted time that I could use to do something else.
- ○ I did not learn anything.
- ○ Other, please tell us...
....

5. Do you want to tell us something else?
....
....

Your Age ....

You are

- ○ Male
- ○ Female

Author details

Annalisa Fogazzi, Fabianna Timelli, Annalisa Vezzoli, Valentina Tradati and Rita Padoan*
Regional Support Cystic Fibrosis Centre, University of Brescia—Children's Hospital, Brescia, Italy

*Address all correspondence to: ritaf54@gmail.com

References

[1] Cox L, Hunt J. Factors that affect adolescents' adherence to diabetes treatment. Nursing Children and Young People. 2015;**27**:16-21

[2] O' Donohoe R, Fullen BM. Adherence of subjects with cystic fibrosis to their home program: A systematic review. Respiratory Care. 2014 Nov;**59**:1731-1746

[3] Retsch-Bogart GZ. Update on new pulmonary therapies. Current Opinion in Pulmonary Medicine. 2009;**15**: 604-610

[4] Bishay LC, S Sawicki GS. Strategies to optimize treatment adherence in adolescent patients with cystic fibrosis. Adolescent Health, Medicine and Therapeutics. 2016;**7**:117-124

[5] Dieninghoff D, Knipel V, Criée CP, Windisch W. Correct inhalation therapy for patients with cystic fibrosis provided by internet-based video clips of the German airway league. Pneumologie. 2015;**69**:583-587

[6] Temme R, Gruber A, Johnson M, Read L, Lu Y, McNamara J. Assessment of parental understanding of positive newborn screening results and carrier status for cystic fibrosis with the use of a short educational video. Journal of Genetic Counseling. 2015;**24**:473-481

Chapter 7

Designing Heterogeneous-mHealth Apps for Cystic Fibrosis Adults

Tamara Vagg, Cathy Shortt, Claire Fleming, Mairead McCarthy, Sabin Tabirca and Barry J. Plant

Abstract

In this chapter, we will discuss the design and development of a patient passport mHealth application for Cystic Fibrosis adults from ideation to app-store release. By allowing the patients access to their own unique data, it is anticipated that it will be of benefit when travelling abroad and between CF centres. The design process followed a pipeline we developed that is informed by patient and healthcare professional input. The app structure resembles an Irish patient file and is divided into three categories: "My CF Info", "My Medical History", and "My Clinical Appointments". My CF Info allows the patient to store personal information such genotype, medical team contact information, physiotherapy, allergies, and medications. My Medical History allows the user to record information such as CF renal disease, CF diabetes, and the insertion/removal of a portacath/gastrostomy tube. My Clinical Appointments allows the user to record the type of appointment (annual assessment, clinic, other) and all information that would ordinarily be inserted into a patient file such as weight, height, spirometry and other comments. Weight and lung function are also displayed in a plot graph. The app has undergone pilot testing with five CF adults before being rolled out onto the Google Play Store.

Keywords: cystic fibrosis, patient passport, mHealth, digital health, self-management

1. Introduction

Cystic Fibrosis (CF) is the most common life limiting genetic disease affecting Caucasians. Patients must adhere to rigorous therapies in order to manage their condition. Such therapies include airway clearance physiotherapy, medications, diet, and exercise.

Ireland has the highest prevalence of CF worldwide, with 1 in 19 people being carriers for the CF gene [1]. Despite this, the life expectancy of patients with CF is rising. A child born with CF in 2009 is now predicted to live into their 50s [2, 3], compared to children born in 1950, of which half would live to the age of 16 and only 3% to 25 years old [4, 5]. However, this increase in life expectancy comes with an increase in patient population. There are now more adult CF patients than pediatric patients in Ireland [6]. It is projected that the pediatric service will need to grow by 25% and the adult service by 75% by 2025 [7]. This growth in adult population and the advent of ICT technologies in the medical space has led to mobile health applications (mHealth apps) being identified as potential powerful tools to assist the growing and ageing CF population in the management of their condition. However, any mHealth app developed in this way must be fully personalisable in order to fit the heterogeneous nature of the treatment and management of CF.

In this chapter we will discuss the design and development of a patient passport mHealth app for CF adults; from ideation to app-store release. This chapter will first begin by introducing the CF unit responsible for its development, before discussing patient passports. Following this, the chapter will introduce the development of this mHealth app which follows the mHealth Design Pipeline as presented by Vagg et al. [8].

1.1 Cork CF multidisciplinary team

CF clinical care is driven by a multidisciplinary team approach. The CF Multidisciplinary Team (MDT) comprises of a mixture of healthcare professionals with varied skill sets to support this multisystem condition. This includes a CF nurse specialist (designated and working full time in CF care), CF physiotherapist (designated and working full time in CF care), and CF dietician (designated and working full time in CF care). The team is supported by a respiratory technician (with a commitment to CF) and psychologist. The MDT is medically-lead by a respiratory specialist with an interest in CF. The respiratory physician/specialist is also supported by a lung-disease research/specialist registrar [9].

The CF MDT at the Cork University Hospital includes: three CF nurse specialists (>30 years collective full time experience in CF care), one dietician (>10 years full time experience in adult and pediatric CF care) one senior physiotherapist (>5 years full time experience CF care), one respiratory technician (>20 years full time experience), and one CF consultant with 10 years as the director of the Cork unit and 10 years' experience in other leading centers both nationally and internationally.

This multidisciplinary team supports the second largest CF center in Ireland with over 180 adult CF patients. The Cork CF multidisciplinary team also lead CFMATTERS; an international multicenter consortium exploring antibiotic therapies in CF [10]. In addition to this, the research team includes a dedicated medical-multimedia research specialist who works directly with the MDT.

1.2 Patient passports definition and review

A patient passport is described by the National Quality Forum (NQF) and Health Service Executive (HSE) as a paper-based system which provides immediate and important information regarding a patient's health or condition to medical professionals [11, 12]. This passport system is implemented for a number of reasons, such as improved patient experience, improving the speed that care is delivered, and as a solution for those patients with learning disabilities [11, 12].

An example of such a passport can be seen for asthma management in the research conducted by Newell et al. [13]. The paper-based passport as presented in this research is developed to store pertinent medical information that an asthmatic would require to receive care on entering an emergency room. Newell et al. found that patients would often experience more fear and stress in this situation as responding medical professionals may ask the patient to repeatedly speak to gain an understanding of this patient's condition, or leave the patient alone so that they can source the information. The paper passport solution is designed to be small and convenient to carry (the size of a credit card) and can provide medical professionals the medical data needed to treat the patient immediately [13]. Another example of these paper-based passports can be seen in the research carried out by Barber et al. [14]. This passport was developed as a medication aid and allowed geriatric patients to record and review their medications and dosages. The researchers found that this system empowered patients to be more in control of their medication and also acted as a mechanism for the patient to communicate and discuss their medications more confidently with their medical team [14].

Patient passports have also been created for other long-term conditions, such as diabetes. Similar to other chronic conditions, diabetic patients must meet with various members of the multidisciplinary healthcare team. For diabetic patients, passports can be beneficial as they allow the patient to record medical data received from each member of the diabetes multidisciplinary team [15]. In this way, passports bridge a communication gap between patients and these various multidisciplinary members [15].

When researching "CF Patient Passports", only two bodies of work were found. The first was a book titled "The Cystic Fibrosis Passport" by Fitzgerald, which aims to aid family members in understanding the needs of children with cystic fibrosis, and to serve as a practical guide to those who care for these children [16]. The second was a quality improvement initiative taken by the Stanford CF Center, which presented a paper-based system that used a passport-sized document containing instructions on how to care for a patient with CF [17]. The document could be presented by a CF patient to a hospital or clinic to ensure the correct measures are taken to avoid potential issues with infection and cross-contamination. Although both passports are important for the care of CF, they do not include features common to long term condition passports as they do not facilitate self-reported medical data that is accessible to patients at all times.

In addition to paper-based CF passports, a search was performed for digital CF patient passports on both the Google Play and iOS mobile App Stores. From this search, only one app was found that allows CF patients to record their medical data, similar to a passport; "CF View" [18]. CFView is an app which was created by "CF Ireland", a CF charity in the Republic of Ireland. The app allows patients to view medical data that has been collected regarding their condition; however, it does not allow patients to enter or save data. In addition to this, CF patients can only use this app if they are part of a CF registry in Ireland, Denmark or Slovenia, and have been issued with an account by that registry. From the findings of the paper based and digital based search, it would appear that there is no freely or publicly available CF patient passport system that allows patients to record basic medical data. Considering the benefits of a patient passport, it can be stipulated that such a tool would be beneficial to adult CF patients.

1.3 Possible issues with patient passports

The previous section outlines cases where patient passports have been used advantageously for patients; asthma patient information, diabetic patient information, medication aid. However, patient passports can also present other challenges which may lead to low adoption rates and minimal impact on patient experience. To investigate this further, Dijkstra et al. interviewed diabetic patients and medical professionals to understand their experience of implementing the passport into their current care system [19]. Concerns expressed by the patients were predominantly focused on security, forgetting the passport, being over encumbered, and need for additional time to enter information into the passport. For security, patients were concerned of the ramifications of losing the passport and the threat this may have on identity theft. Furthermore, some paper passports can be the size of a small A5 copy and cannot fit into a pocket easily. For this reason, patients expressed concerns with forgetting to bring the passport to clinical appointments and also friends or work colleagues seeing or finding the passport. As for time, patients felt that entering information into the passport could often take away from the valuable time they had with their healthcare team [19].

When interviewing medical professionals Dijkstra et al. found that often there was no clear agenda for the passport and how it would be of benefit to patient self-management. Consequently, it was unclear at which stage a passport should be introduced formally to a patient to ensure they know how to use it sufficiently. Moreover, there are discrepancies over who is responsible to manage the passport, if it is of benefit to medical professionals, and how this passport can be implemented seamlessly to the current healthcare system [19].

2. Patient mHealth survey

The General mHealth Design Pipeline [8] first suggests gathering insights from key stakeholders to mHealth applications (patients and medical professionals). As such a survey is conducted with CF adult patients from the Cork University Hospital to include their insights before developing a written report with medical professionals. To evaluate if CF adults would find an mHealth app beneficial and to determine what aspect of patient education and patient management that is of interest to CF adult patients, an 18-part multiple choice survey was created and validated over a series of three formal meetings with the Cork CF multidisciplinary (see appendix). Participation in this survey was voluntary, and the inclusion criteria for this survey were that participants were 18 years old or older and owned a smartphone. Surveys were offered to all patients attending their designated outpatient appointment over a 4 week period at the CF Day Ward in Cork University Hospital. Ethical approval for this survey is obtained via the Clinical Research Ethics Committee in University College Cork. During the study period, 49 eligible patients completed the survey; no patients opted-not to complete the survey. The collected survey data was anonymized, and the only clinical information collected in this survey was that the participants have CF and are attending the Cork CF center.

2.1 Survey results

A total of 49 completed surveys were analyzed. Of the 49 participants, 55% of respondents use an Android smartphone and 40% use an iPhone. It was reported that 38% of participants have a mHealth app installed on their smartphone device such as exercise trackers or calorie counters; however, only 10% (n = 5) know of or are aware of an app which targets CF. Those CF focused mHealth apps identified by the participants are "CF MedCare", "MyFitnessPal", "CFMATTERS STUDY INFO", and "CF View". Two of the five participants reported having a CF app installed on their phone (CF View and CF MedCare). The remaining 44 participants who do not know of any CF apps or have a CF app installed were then asked to explain their answer. Of the 44 participants, 20 patients reported being unaware of the existence of CF apps; *"I don't think there is one"*, and three advised that they are not interested in a CF app; *"Not Interested"*.

The participants are also given the option to choose multiple aspects of their CF that they would like targeted by a CF mHealth app. To note, the participants could choose as many of these options as applicable. It was found that

"New Research Developments" (55%), "Medication" (55%), and "Physiotherapy" (47.5%) are the areas of most interest to the participants, followed by "Diet" (42.50%), "Monitoring" (40%), "Social Networks" (40%), "Self-Psychological Help" (37.50%), "News" (32.50%), "Education" (27.50%), and "Management" (20%). One patient reported *"None"* for this question.

Further questions were presented regarding specific features within mHealth applications. 85% of participants agreed that they would like to receive notifications from the app, such as reminders to take medication or next clinical appointment. When asked would the participant play a game to support their CF, the results were more dispersed; 32.65% agreed they would play a game, 34.69% reported they would not and 30.61% were unsure. Ten of the 49 participants reported as being part of a clinical trial currently or in the past. Six of these 10 participants reported that an mHealth application would have been of use to this trial for data collection or self-reporting.

A series of questions regarding the collection of personal medical data was then presented. When asked if their CF medical information, such as genotype and medical history, is difficult to remember, 32.65% of participants regarded this information as difficult and 42% regarded this information as easy to remember. 26.5% of participants agreed they would record their medical information in a mHealth app. 46.9% agreed they would store this information if the mHealth app is password protected and 16% (n = 8) agreed they would if the mHealth app is password protected and does not have access to the internet. One participant reported being unsure to recording their medical data. Each participant was then given the option to further explain their reasoning for choosing their security preference. These results are listed below.

- *Yes: If password protected*
    - *"Security is priority"*
    - *"Only available to me and no online servers"*
    - *"Privacy Matters"*
    - *"As long as it is stored on a secure database"*
- *Yes: If password protected and does not connect to the internet*
    - *"It would be very helpful/useful to store the data for myself but I would be cautious about who else could access it"*
    - *"It is personal information and so it would need to be very secure"*
    - *"It is personal and private info"*
- *Unsure*
    - *"Security Issue"*

To note, two additional answers were submitted for "*Yes: If password protected*"; however, these answers were specific to the perceived usefulness of such an mHealth application and not their rationale for their security preference and hence negated from the above list. The two submitted answers include: "*Handy if required when travelling/emergencies*" and "*It would help to track what might have been working at the time to maintain lung function (e.g. meds/physio)*". In a follow up question specific to the usefulness of such an application, 87.5% of participants reported that they would find it beneficial to have access to their medical data through an mHealth app. Of the 49 participants 67.35% agreed that an mHealth app that recorded their medical data would be useful and 61.22% confirmed they would use an app to record this data.

Two questions were also posed regarding travel and admission to the accident and emergency department in a hospital to determine scenarios in which the recording of medical information would be of benefit (similar to other passports as discussed earlier). 75.5% of participants reported having gone travelling outside of Ireland and only 12 participants have had to visit a hospital emergency room due their CF. When the participants were asked if they would use a CF mHealth app if created, 67.5% said yes; however, 27.5% were unsure.

Lastly, the participants were given the option to share what they felt a CF mHealth app should target. Twenty three participants suggested mHealth apps which can be categorized under three headings; Management, Support, and Information. Sixteen participants suggested management apps to track and store their medical information to aid in self-management of the condition. Examples of this category include *"Medication taken/taking"* and *"Medical Info i.e weight lung fx exercise + diet plans"*. Six participants suggested apps that can access medical information such as drug names and new treatments or research. An example of this category includes *"Proper medical names of meds"* and *"New treatments"*. Lastly, five participants suggest apps which can allow for support among CF patients, similar to social networks; *"Experience/Information sharing between other patients"*.

2.2 Survey discussion

It is noted that slightly more patients own an Android device; however, the number of iPhone owners was still high. The first observation to note from the survey results is the paucity in awareness of CF apps. Only five patients reported being aware of CF mHealth apps, and only two patients have these apps installed. To note one of the apps, "MyFitnessPal", which was regarded as a CF specific mHealth app, is not. This app does not target any specific cohort and includes personalisable goal setting, such as weight gain, weight loss, weight maintenance. When questioned further this seemed to be primarily due to being unaware of such apps; *"I don't think there is any"*. However, despite this lack of awareness, the CF adult participants still demonstrated interest and expectations on what a CF app should focus on. New Research Developments, Medication, and Physiotherapy focused apps were of the most interest to these participants. Additionally, tracking medical data and receiving alerts or reminders were the most popular features.

It is important to note that the participants demonstrated concerns regarding data security and as such any mHealth app created for these patients will need to be fully transparent *i.e* full disclosure on what data is being collected, who is it being used/viewed by, and the security measures in place.

Personalizing educational content in this way is synonymous with patient management mechanisms and interventions, as the multimedia is educating the patient on their medical condition data or personal symptoms. Examples of patient management interventions include: audio tapes, booklets, patient credit card/patient passports, counseling, exercise sessions, individual plan/goal setting, manuals, videos, and lectures/talks [20].

3. App design

3.1 Considerations from similar passports

The issues with patient passports, as listed in the Section 1.3, pertain to diabetes passports only; however, these problems are transferable. As such, they have been considered in the design of the adult cystic fibrosis passport. Firstly, by deploying the CF passport as a mobile app a number of these pitfalls may be resolved. When considering the concerns the patients expressed for security and the possibility of identity theft, an mHealth passport can be secured via a username and password. Furthermore, if the phone was lost or stolen, all passport data will be encrypted and not easily accessible. As the passport will be in a digital form on a smartphone, issues regarding the patient being over encumbered or finding it difficult to carry the passport on their person are removed. Furthermore, as the data entered into the mHealth passport is minimal, there will be no smartphone memory usage issues. Finally, as the passport will be in an mHealth form, it is unlikely that a patient will forget their smartphone and subsequently reduces the risk of forgetting the passport at clinical appointments.

3.2 Considerations from MDT meeting

The remaining issues, as highlighted by members of the diabetes healthcare team, were discussed with cystic fibrosis nurse specialists at the Cork University Hospital. The below discussed solutions were work shopped and agreed upon by consensus before being implemented into the app design. Firstly, identifying the point of care the app should be introduced was considered. In the current healthcare model, the passport shall be introduced to patients who have just transferred from pediatric to the adult orientated facility. However, the app can also be introduced to existing adult patients. During this introduction, a CF nurse specialist will explain the aim of this app and why it will be of use to the patient, the data that can be entered into the passport, and when/how to use this app when meeting members of their healthcare team. The nurse will then assist the patient in entering data that can help set up their profile in the app (e.g. contact information for their healthcare team, genotype). The patient will then be made aware that all data entered into the app is voluntary and cannot be viewed outside the app. The nurse will also explain to the patient that the patient is responsible for entering data into the app.

Finally, concerns surrounding time to enter information into the passport was discussed. In Ireland, An adult CF clinic appointment can last approximately 1 hour and 15 minutes. During this clinic, patients meet each member of the MDT. The first member of this team is a CF nurse specialist who will encourage the patient to enter the data into their passport while the nurse enters the data into their patient file. Between meeting each member of the MDT there is approximately 15 minutes of free time. Therefore, if similar to the diabetic patients, the CF patients feel as though they would prefer to spend the time with the medical team member, they can enter the information during this free time instead.

Considering the benefits of a patient passport and the patient insight provided by the Patient mHealth Survey, it can be stipulated that such a tool would be beneficial to adult CF patients. Hence, this research will develop and evaluate a patient passport targeted at adults with cystic fibrosis. However, unlike the aforementioned passports, the proposed passport will be developed as a mobile application. The agenda for this app is to provide CF adults with their basic medical information and also to allow them to record their medications, along with medical data from clinical appointments. In doing this, adult CF patients may become more aware of their condition and symptoms. Additionally, three scenarios have been identified in which the proposed app may be of use to a CF adult. Firstly, it can allow a patient to receive immediate care when travelling abroad. Secondly, it will allow patients to receive care if travelling between adult CF centers. Lastly, it can be used to communicate between healthcare team members. These scenarios and the design of the passport app with reference to the General mHealth Design Pipeline will be discussed further in the following section.

4. General mHealth design pipeline overview

This section will discuss the design and development of the app under the headings Preparation, Back-End, Front-End, and Deployment, in accordance to the mHealth Design Pipeline described by Vagg et al. [8]. To note, a series of informal scoping meetings was held with the CF nurse specialists from the Cork adult CF unit (>10). Post initial development a further formal meeting with the entire CF multidisciplinary team was held to sign off on the CF passport app.

4.1 Preparation

Before developing or designing the CF Patient Passport, the app's purpose, app type, ethics, and regulations are defined. These considerations are discussed and outlined in the proceeding sub-sections.

4.1.1 Purpose

This section will discuss the components necessary to create a written report before developing the app. Firstly and agenda for the mHealth passport is outlined, so that the app can be implemented into the current health care model and have a positive impact on the patient. Identifying the proposed agenda of the app was discussed with members to serve the patient were identified and are listed below.

Scenario 1 Traveling between CF centers: In Ireland, there are five CF focused centers. Patients can transfer between these centers for varying medical or personal reasons. However, as patient data is stored as a hardcopy, there may be a delay between the patient arriving at the center and the medical professional accessing their clinical data. In this scenario, the mHealth passport can ensure that the patient can provide their basic medical data when arriving to the new unit. Such information can include recent lung function history, medications, allergies, genotypes.

Scenario 2 Travelling abroad: As quality of life and survival rates increase, more and more CF patients are travelling abroad. In this scenario if the patient would require any medical care when travelling abroad, the mHealth passport would ensure that the patient could provide their basic medical data (and contact information for their healthcare team) to the attending medical professional.

Scenario 3 Bridging Gaps between the healthcare team: In Ireland, it can be approximately 3–4 months between clinical appointments in the adult unit. Between appointments, patients may visit a General Practitioner (GP) and begin an antibiotic treatment and this data must be entered into their patient file at their next clinical appointment. The details of the new antibiotics can be either forgotten, or only partially remembered. In this scenario the app can record any interaction with any member of their health care team as well as new prescriptions or changes to care to provide a broader view of their care.

It is anticipated that the app will be first offered to CF adolescents transferring to adult care. However, it can also be suggested to any CF adult. The app will be made available on both iOS app store and Google Play store, in addition to being made available on the Cork Hospital CF Centre web page. Patients will be given time during clinical appointments to enter the data with the CF nurse specialists, or they can enter the data during non-contact time.

All data collected through the app will be stored locally on the device. It shall not be transmitted or viewed by any other personnel. The data recorded will not be analyzed; however, some data shall be visualized in two interactive graphs. The first graph will display Weight over time, and the second will display lung function as FVC% and FEV1%. An example of this graph can be seen in **Figure 1**. The graph is interactive and can allow users to touch different points on the plot to view its corresponding information. The user can also save reminders for clinical appointments or take medications through the app.

4.1.2 Application type

The proposed CF Patient Passport can be considered as both an In Vitro app and a Wellbeing/Lifestyle app. The passport is intended to record a patient's basic medical information and simultaneously plot data on a graph; as such, it is considered an In Vitro app. It is not considered a Medical Device, as this data is not being used to perform a diagnostic or any immediate decision making for the patient.

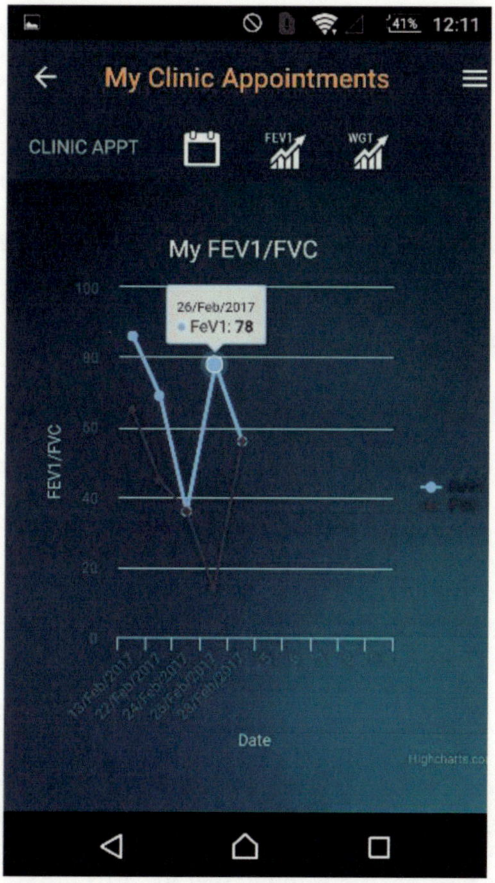

Figure 1.
Lung function (FEV1, FVC) in "My Clinic Appointments".

However, it can also be considered as a Wellbeing/Lifestyle app as it may improve health behaviors among this cohort as they become more aware of their own medical data/symptoms.

4.1.3 Ethics and regulations

All evaluations performed with patients received ethical approval from the Clinical Research Ethics Committee in Cork. The app is currently available on the Google Play store in Ireland and is GDPR compliant.

4.2 Back-end

To ensure that the app can be deployed to both Android and iOS, Cordova PhoneGap [21] was used to develop the mHealth passport. PhoneGap uses web technologies such as HTML, CSS, and JavaScript in addition to Frameworks for navigations and layouts. For this passport, Framework 7 [22] is incorporated into the app to ensure a consistent layout/style across both Android and iOS. The language and dialogue used in the app is simple so that it can be understood by non-medical persons. All graphs are developed using the Highcharts.js framework [23]. This section will discuss the validation of content and dialogue within the application before discussing the data that can be recorded via the passport app.

4.2.1 Content and dialogue validation

As CF is a genetic disease, patients have grown up listening to and using medical terminology to aid in the management of their condition. Therefore, the medical data that can be recorded in the app is familiar to this cohort; however, the manner in which the data is requested may be new to these patients, and subsequently may require validation. A meeting was held with CF nurse specialists to discuss the instructions on how to enter data in the app. The CF Nurse specialists were enlisted for this task due to their extensible knowledge in communicating with this cohort. There is no imagery used within the app, however, there are two proposed graphs. The graphs and app instruction were modified until validation from the nurse specialists was given.

4.2.2 Data information requirements

As the data are not being transferred and viewed by other personnel, an opt-out service and DPA policy was not required in the app. As the CF Patient Passport was developed as part of a pilot study, information pertaining to all intentions of what data was to be collected and how it was then stored was provided to patients in a participant information sheet. It was anticipated that once the app was made available via app stores and over the web, these intentions would also need to be listed.

4.2.3 Data and data analysis

Focusing on the outlined scenarios (travelling between centers, traveling abroad, and bridging the gap between the healthcare team) a meeting was held with the CF MDT to discuss which data should be recorded in the app to fulfill these objectives. From this meeting it was found that the mHealth passport should follow the same architecture as a patient file. In Ireland, a patient file can include information stored once (genotype, date of birth, genotype *etc.*), information that can sometimes be recorded (such as new medical conditions or procedures), and lastly data that is recorded at every clinical appointment (lung function, weight, height *etc.*). Therefore the mHealth passport is separated into three core sections and described below. To note, all data entered into the passport can be edited or deleted if desired. These sections can be seen in **Figure 2** (right).

Section 1 My CF Information: This section is targeted at the information in the patient file that are only recorded once. This data generally describes a patient profile such as date of diagnosis, genotype, sweat test results, allergies, contact numbers for the healthcare team, and allergies. This can be seen in **Figure 3** (left).

Section 2 My Medical History: This section is dedicated to the occasional data and is divided into two sections. "My Medical Procedures" and "My Medical Conditions". The first section is targeted towards procedures a CF patients may have undergone such as the insertion of a gastrostomy tube, or the removal of a portacath. The second section focuses on new conditions or diseases which may have developed, such as diabetes.

Section 3 My Clinic Appointments: The final section records data that are entered into a patient file at each clinical appointment. This data can include Blood Pressure (BP), weight, height, date, lung function (FEV1% and FVC%), bugs in mucus, new treatments. This section can also be used for phone calls with the healthcare team, GP Visits, and annual assessment.

4.2.4 Security operations

As the data is being stored on the smartphone, security precautions are put in place for local storage. First, the mHealth app is password protected (as seen in **Figure 2** left). In the event of a forgotten password, a randomly generated password is created within the app and emailed to the user. All data stored in the CF Patient Passport is optional. Any data that is recorded is encrypted using the Advanced Encryption Standard (AES) algorithm and stored in a local SQLite database. If the app is uninstalled from the device, the databases will also be deleted.

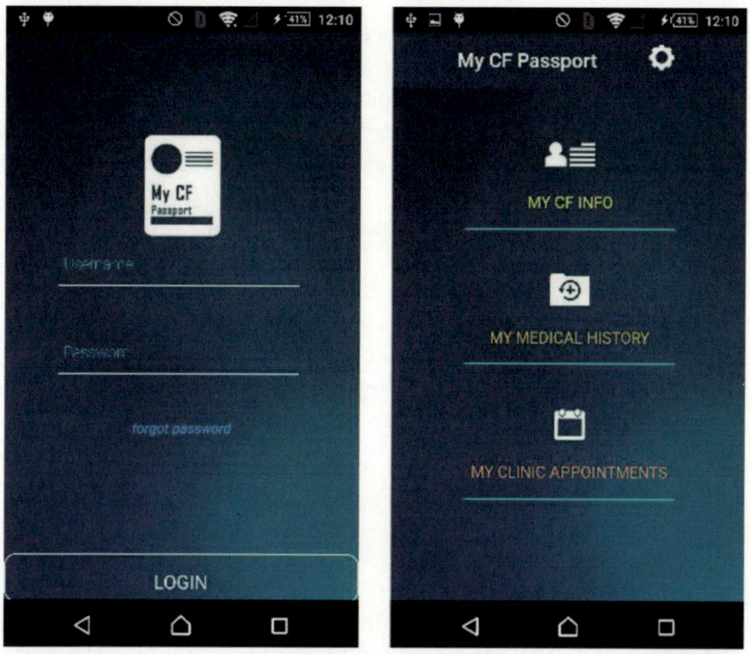

Figure 2.
Login screen (left) and main menu in the passport (right).

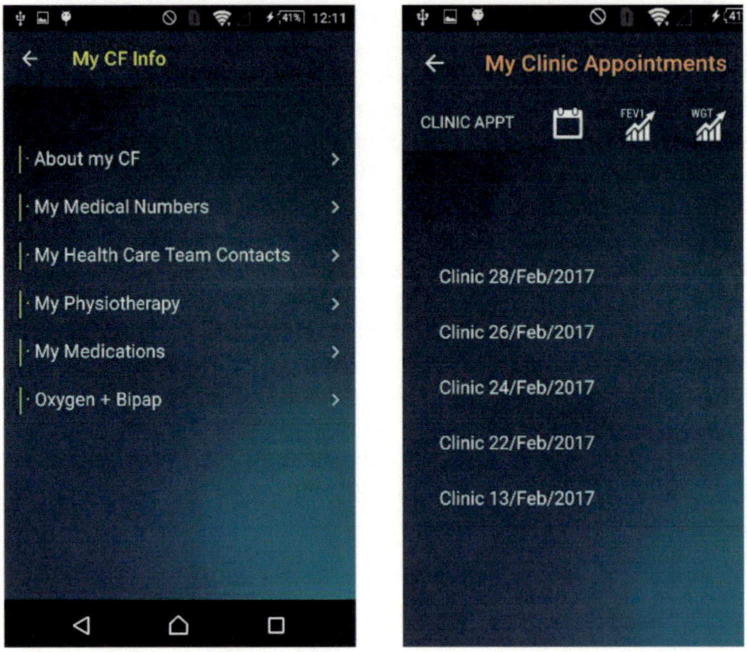

Figure 3.
Menu from the "My CF Info" section (left) and list of saved clinical appointments in "My Clinic Appointments" (right).

4.3 Front-end

In keeping with the mHealth pipeline discussed previously, the User Interface (UI) and User Experience (UX) of the app are discussed.

4.3.1 User interface (UI)

A meeting was held with CF nurse specialists and physiotherapists to discuss the plausibility of an Adaptive UI. From this meeting it was determined that a UI model was not required. It was considered that perhaps an Adaptive Navigation model may be beneficial for the use cases as described in 6.5.1 under Preparation; however, this was later dismissed as data recorded and shown in the app is at the patient's discretion.

Informal discussions between the CF nurse specialists and the CF adults attending clinic found that this cohort would prefer the UI to be designed so that it does not appear to be a mHealth app. As such, the icon that was to appear on the main screen of the user's smartphone does not contain any indications that the app is for CF; hence this icon is named "My Passport". Furthermore, the style and UI elements in the app were designed so that they do not appear to be "medical" or "clinical". Similarly, all menus and buttons were created to reflect the data collected.

4.3.2 User experience (UX)

On reviewing diabetic patient passports, a number of issues which could prevent the use of such of an intervention was found. Of interest to the UX aspects of this mHealth app is outlining how the app should be implemented into the current care system. A solution for this is discussed in Section 3.2. It is agreed by CF nurse specialists that the app will be offered to CF adolescents transferring to CF adult care and CF adults already registered in the hospital. If the patients are interested in using the app a workshop will be given by nurses on how to use the app and the data that can be recorded. The nurses will then assist the patient in entering any historical and profile data. Time is then allocated during clinical visits for patients to enter this data with a CF nurse or during non-contact time.

4.4 Deployment

In this section, further testing and reviews conducted on the app are discussed. Following on from the results of the reviews and testing, future plans for the deployment of this mHealth app are outlined.

4.4.1 Stress test

The purpose of this test was to evaluate the performance of this app and its design. Seven participants without CF were enlisted who all owned Android devices. The decision to recruit non-CF participants was intended to identify performance and design issues and to remedy them. For the stress test, participants from a similar age range to the target CF adult cohort were chosen. Five participants (three females and two males) between 19 and 51 were recruited. The technical capability of this participants varied, some participants were novices at using technology, while others were ICT professionals.

The participants were asked to download the mHealth passport onto their smartphones and test for 3 months. During this time participants were required to enter, edit, and delete data to "My CF Information" and "My Medical History" a minimum of once a month. However, they were requested perform the same tasks in the "My Clinic Appointments" more frequently (once a week). Each month the participants sent a report of any issues they encountered using the app (such as performance, usability, or general feedback) via email.

At the end of this stress test it was found that there were no major performance issues and the users did not find the mHealth passport difficult to use. The primary issue reported on was a style issue that occurred on different phone screen resolutions whereby the submit button to enter data would remain behind the keyboard (users must close the keyboard before being able to submit). Another issue reported was the lack of clarity or structure when entering dates into the mHealth app. The final issue reported on was that the default "Go" button on the smartphone keyboard did not move to the next text field as expected. Following this feedback, the styling was adjusted and retested on different devices to ensure the submit button was no longer hidden, a calendar was implemented to enter in the date, and finally functionality was created and bound to the "Go" button to ensure users could navigate through the form items. The above solutions were implemented in preparation for pilot testing with CF adult patients.

4.4.2 Peer review

The CF Patient Passport was then presented to CF nurse specialists, CF physiotherapists and respiratory consultants for review. During this review, the app purpose, aesthetics, dialogue, content, and functionality was reviewed. Slight modifications are recommended by the reviewers to improve the quality of data entered and prevent errors. Examples of this feedback included the incorporation of a drop-down menu which contains all possible bugs that can be growing in mucus as opposed to the patient manually entering this data. Similarly, in places where patients must enter a date range (*e.g.* start date and end date) it should be possible for the user to enter just a month and year as opposed to date, month, and year. Overall it is agreed that the CF patient passport can be of benefit to CF adult patients as it will allow for this cohort to always have access to their basic medical data and become more aware of their own condition and symptoms.

4.4.3 Patient review

Following on from the stress test and peer review, ethical approval was granted by the Clinical Research Ethics Committee in the University College Cork for pilot testing with CF adults from the Cork University Hospital. The inclusion criteria for this study was that patients must be 18 years old or older and own an Android smartphone. Participation in this study was voluntary and was offered to patients during clinical appointments over two consecutive days. Five eligible patients were identified and recruited by the CF nurse specialists. All five patients agreed to partake in the study; one participant was female and the remaining four were male. Each participant was provided with an information sheet outlining the purpose of the app, the data collected, intentions for the data, and security measures. After the app was installed on their devices, the participants partook in a short workshop with the CF nurse specialists, who demonstrated how to use the app. The CF nurse specialists also assisted the participants in entering any of their historical or patient file data into the passport app. The patients were then asked to test the app over 3 months before completing a feedback questionnaire, which was provided to them at their next closest clinical appointment.

5. Results

During the three-month study period, one male participant lost his smartphone and as such was unable to complete the feedback questionnaire. Of the remaining four participants, three reported their smartphone models: a Oneplus 5, Sony Xperia M5, and Samsung Galaxy. All four participants agreed that they were provided with sufficient information to use the app. The participants were then asked to rate the appearance of the app from 1 to 5 (1 being Do not Like It, 3 being Neutral, and 5 being Like It), with two participants rating the app a 3 and the remaining participants rating the appearance a 4.

During the study period all participants reported inserting data into the app. Two participants confirmed they used the app to share their medical information. When asked to explain this further, one participant reported using the app in a clinical appointment. When asked to rate the difficulty of the app from 1 to 5 (1 being Difficult, 3 being Moderate, and 5 being Easy), one participant rated the app a 5, two participants rated the app a 4, and the remaining participant rated the app a 3. When asked which parts of the app was difficult, the participant who rated the app a 3 reported difficulty in inputting "some information". One other participant also advised that the built-in back button on their device caused the app to close instead of returning to the previous page and was therefore reliant on the built-in navigation bar. When asked which features the participant would like to remove from the app, three participants reported none. When asked what features the participant would like to add to the app, one participant advised they would like for their doctor to be able to access the data or input new data remotely.

The participants were next asked to rate the helpfulness of the app from 1 to 5 (1 being Not Helpful, 3 Indifferent, and 5 being Helpful). One participant reported a 5 for this question, two reported a 4, and one participant reported a 3. When asked to explain their answer, the participant who reported a 3 did not elaborate further. However, two other participants remarked that the app is helpful as it allows them access to their medical information:

"It's useful to have this information in an easily accessible place"
"It's handy for me to have my information so readily accessible"

This is further enforced in Question 10, where all participants agreed that it was beneficial to have access to their basic medical information through the app. When asked who the participants believe is responsible for inputting data into the app, three participants reported that the responsibility is theirs, while one participant believed it was the shared responsibility of the participant and their CF treatment team. The users were then asked to explain their answer. It was found from these answers that users believe it is their responsibility as entering data should be at their discretion. However, one participant welcomes guidance from their healthcare team.

"I put what I think is necessary"
"Personal info on a personal device should only be entered by the owner unless explicit permission is given. I think I am ultimately responsible for knowing about my condition and recording the information but I might not always know the most important information to be recorded which is why my nurses and doctors should also have input."
"It's my app and on my phone, so it's my own responsibility to keep it updated"

One participant reported a barrier which prevented the editing of data. This participant found that some saved data in the My CF Info section of the app could not be edited, and instead needed to be deleted and inputted again, which they regarded as frustrating. The participants were then asked to rate the regularity of using the app from 1 to 5 (1 being Not Regularly, 3 being Sometimes, and 5 being Regularly). Two participants rated this question a 1, one participant reported a 3, and the remaining participant reported a 4. When asked to list scenarios in which they felt the app maybe useful, the participants reported the following scenarios:

"If I got sick on holidays could show what I'm on"
"Listing medication/medical details at clinics etc"
"Sharing information with my GP or if I'm traveling and need to share information with a doctor. Going abroad or another hospital/GP"

It can be seen from the above scenarios that participants felt that the app maybe of most benefit when travelling abroad or sharing information with medical and healthcare professionals. Lastly, the participants were asked to rate how adequate the security precautions within the app are from 1 to 5 (1 being not adequate and 5 being adequate), to which two participants rated a 5, and the remaining two rated a 4.

5.1 Initial observations

It is acknowledged that some limitations of this study are the small number of participants and the disproportionate ratio of male to female participants, which could present a potential gender bias. There was a notable difference in the participants reported regularity of the apps use. Patients were asked about how often they would use the app. At face value, not regularly could be perceived as concerning; however, CF patients attend CF clinic appointments quarterly, and entering data is at the patient's discretion. In addition to this, minor issues in device functionality were reported by this cohort, which have since been addressed and resolved.

Interestingly, unlike the findings of the paper-based patient passport, participants of this study identified themselves as the sole or major inputter of data. This is perhaps a clear advantage to paper-based passports, which reported uncertainties in this responsibility, as discussed previously. This may be attributed to the passport being based on a patient's personal device, as opposed being provided to them in a hospital branded booklet.

Moreover, the app in its current form was received positively by the participants of this study. All participants agreed that having access to their basic medical information is of benefit to them. Furthermore, these patients envision practical scenarios in which this app may be of benefit to them in the future.

6. Conclusion and future works

The app is currently available for free on the Google Play Irish store. Future works would include deploying the app to iOS app store and being linked to the Cork CF Centre website. Information pertaining to data usage intentions and storage will is made available on the app store description page. The results of the patient survey conducted found that this cohort showed interest in the recording and viewing of their medical data in a convenient and manageable way. To this end, it was found that the concept of a patient passport could prove to be a suitable solution. Patient passports have been proven to help patients with self-management as it facilitates the ability to closely monitor their own condition. Hence a passport application was developed so that CF adults could record their medications and basic CF information. It is also anticipated that this will allow these patients to receive care when travelling between centers and abroad. A pilot study with four participants demonstrates that CF adults perceive this passport app to be beneficial as it allows them access to their basic medical information. It was also found through the pilot study that participants would not use this mHealth app frequently. This is a similar finding to paper-based passports, as patients only enter the data into the app during clinical appointments (quarterly) and share data in specific scenarios such as with a GP, or when travelling abroad. As the app is password protected, the user must be able to enter in their correct credentials and navigate through the app to share data. However, in situations such as needing to attend the accident and emergency room, this may cause further frustration to the patient, whereas a paper-based passport can be handed to medical professional who can locate all data needed in order to provide care. This is perhaps one advantage of the paper-based system over the digital mHealth app. To contend with this, future iterations of the app may include a Generate PDF button on the main menu which will compile all the most pertinent medical data into an A4 PDF which can be shown to medical professionals via the device or emailed to them directly. This suggestion can also be applied to mHealth patient passports for other conditions. It is also noted that the data from the app is stored locally only. For this reason if the phone became lost or stolen, it would not be possible to restore a profile onto a new phone, in this case the user would have to re-input all their data. This design choice was made based on the feedback from the mHealth survey regarding security and the app connecting to other online sources. However, future iterations of this app will implement the ability to migrate data from one smartphone to another in the event the user purchases a new phone. Once the data has been migrated, data stored on the old smartphone device will be deleted. In conclusion, an mHealth patient passport is desirable among the adult CF cohort and we believe it can have significant impact on how patients can manage their condition and have access to their data.

Acknowledgements

We would like to acknowledge funding from CFMATTERS which is funded under the European Union's Seventh Framework Programme (FP7/2007–2013) under grant agreement no 603038.

Conflict of interest

There is no conflicts of interest.

Author details

Tamara Vagg[1,2,3*], Cathy Shortt[2], Claire Fleming[2], Mairead McCarthy[2], Sabin Tabirca[1] and Barry J. Plant[2,3]

1 Department of Computer Science, University College Cork, Cork, Ireland

2 Cork Adult CF Centre, Cork University Hospital, University College Cork, Cork, Ireland

3 CRF-C, HRB Clinical Research Facility, Cork, Ireland

*Address all correspondence to: tv3@cs.ucc.ie

References

[1] Farrell P, Joffe S, Foley L, Canny GJ, Mayne P, Rosenberg M. Diagnosis of cystic fibrosis in the Republic of Ireland: Epidemiology and costs. Irish Medical Journal. 2007;**100**(8):557-560

[2] MacKenzie T, Gifford AH, Sabadosa KA, Quinton HB, Knapp EA, Goss CH, et al. Longevity of patients with cystic fibrosis in 2000 to 2010 and beyond: Survival analysis of the Cystic Fibrosis Foundation patient registry. Annals of Internal Medicine. 2014;**161**(4):233-241. DOI: 10.7326/M13-0636

[3] McIntyre K. Gender and survival in cystic fibrosis. Current Opinion in Pulmonary Medicine. 2013;**19**(6): 692-697. DOI: 10.1097/MCP. 0b013e328365af49

[4] Dodge JA, Lewis PA, Stanton M, Wilsher J. Cystic fibrosis mortality and survival in the UK: 1947–2003. The European Respiratory Journal. 2007; **29**(3):522-526. DOI: 10.1183/ 09031936.00099506

[5] Barben J, Castellani C, Dankert-Roelse J, Gartner S, Kashirskaya N, Linnane B, et al. The expansion and performance of national newborn screening programmes for cystic fibrosis in Europe. Journal of Cystic Fibrosis. 2017;**16**(2):207-213. DOI: 10.1016/j. jcf.2016.12.012

[6] O'Sullivan BP, Freedman SD. Cystic fibrosis. Lancet. 2009;**373**(9678): 1891-1904. DOI: 10.1016/S0140-6736 (09)60327-5

[7] Burgel PR, Bellis G, Olesen HV, Viviani L, Zolin A, Blasi F, et al. Future trends in cystic fibrosis demography in 34 European countries. The European Respiratory Journal. 2015;**46**(1):133-141. DOI: 10.1183/09031936.00196314

[8] Vagg T, Plant BJ, Tabirca S. A general mhealth design pipeline. In: Proceedings of the 14th International Conference on Advances in Mobile Computing and Multi Media (MoMM 16); November 2016. Singapore: ACM; 2016. pp. 190-194. DOI: 10.1145/ 3007120.3007147

[9] Conway S, Balfour-Lynn IM, De Rijcke K, Drevinek P, Foweraker J, Havermans T, et al. European Cystic Fibrosis Society Standards of Care: Framework for the cystic fibrosis centre. Journal of Cystic Fibrosis. 2014;**13**: S3-S22. DOI: 10.1016/j.jcf.2014.03.009

[10] CFMATTERS. CFMATTERS Home [Internet]. 2014. Available at: https:// www.cfmatters.eu/ [Accessed: 05 October 2017]

[11] National Quality Forum. Patient Passport Encourages Better Engagement with Providers [Internet]. 2014. Available at: http://www.qualityforum. org/Patient_Passport.aspx [Accessed: 25 July 2017]

[12] Health Service Executive. Hospital Passport for Patients with a Communication Difficulty [Internet]. Available at: http://www.hse.ie/eng/about/Who/ONMSD/Practicedevelopment/Practice%20Development%20Innovations/Acute%20PD%20Innovations/Hospital%20Passport%20for%20Patients%20with%20a%20Communication%20Difficulty.html [Accessed: 25 July 2017]

[13] Newell K, Basi T, Hume S. Development of a patient passport in asthma management. Nursing Standard. 2014;**29**(7):37-42. DOI: 10.7748/ ns.29.7.37.e8970

[14] Barber S, Thakkar K, Marvin V, Franklin BD, Bell D. evaluation of my medication passport: A patient-completed aide-memoire designed by patients, for patients, to help towards medicines optimisation. BMJ Open. 2014;**4**(8):e005608. DOI: 10.1136/ bmjopen-2014-005608

[15] Simmons D, Gamble GD, Foote S, Cole DR, Coster G. The New Zealand diabetes passport study: A randomized controlled trial of the impact of a diabetes passport on risk factors for diabetes-related complications. Diabetic Medicine. 2004;**21**(3):214-217

[16] Fitzgerald DA. A Cystic Fibrosis Passport. Mawson ACT: Clareville Press; 2013

[17] Lucile Packard Children's Hospital Stanford. Cystic Fibrosis Center News [Internet]. 2015. Available at: http://med.stanford.edu/content/dam/sm/cfcenter/documents/facts/LPCH.CF.NL.Spring2015.lores.pdf [Accessed: 25 July 2017]

[18] OpenApp. CF View [Internet]. 2017. Available at: https://play.google.com/store/apps/details?id=com.openapp.cfview&hl=en [Accessed: 25 July 2017]

[19] Dijkstra R, Braspenning J, Grol R. Empowering patients: How to implement a diabetes passport in hospital care. Patient Education and Counseling. 2002;**47**(2):173-177

[20] Barlow J, Wright C, Sheasby J, Turner A, Hainsworth J. Self-management approaches for people with chronic conditions: A review. Patient Education and Counseling. 2002;**48**(2):177-187

[21] Adobe Systems Inc. Adobe PhoneGap [Internet]. 2011–2017. Available at: http://phonegap.com/ [Accessed: 25 July 2017]

[22] iDangero.us. Framework7 [Internet]. 2016–2017. Available at: https://framework7.io/, 2016–2017 [Accessed: 25 July 2017]

[23] HighSoft. High Charts [Internet]. 2009–2017. Available at: http://www.highcharts.com/, 2009–2017 [Accessed: 25 July 2017]